YOUR KNOWLEDGE HAS VALUE

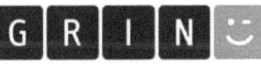

Bibliographic information published by the German National Library:

The German National Library lists this publication in the National Bibliography; detailed bibliographic data are available on the Internet at http://dnb.dnb.de .

Imprint:

Copyright © 2017 GRIN Verlag
Print and binding: Books on Demand GmbH, Norderstedt Germany
ISBN: 9783346135919

This book at GRIN:

https://www.grin.com/document/538444

Tarannum Rahman

Cognitive and Behavioral Effects of Music Therapy on Older Adults with Dementia

GRIN Verlag

GRIN - Your knowledge has value

Since its foundation in 1998, GRIN has specialized in publishing academic texts by students, college teachers and other academics as e-book and printed book. The website www.grin.com is an ideal platform for presenting term papers, final papers, scientific essays, dissertations and specialist books.

Visit us on the internet:

http://www.grin.com/

http://www.facebook.com/grincom

http://www.twitter.com/grin_com

A Systematic Review of Cognitive and Behavioral Effect of Music Therapy on Older Adults

With Dementia

PH 7013: Research Dissertation

TARANNUM RAHMAN

10/30/2017

Total Word Count (Date: 28 Aug 2017):

15,000 words in total (excluding references and appendices)

Table of Contents

ACKNOWLEDGEMENT

It is a great opportunity for me to write about the subject like 'Dementia', where the scope of research is still available. At the time of the study period, I had tried my heart and soul to go through different books, articles, journals, websites like CINAHL, Psych Info, Hinari, PubMed, Google scholars and so forth; which helped me to get acquainted with this topic. I am focusing on those specific topics, which are important for us for further resource allocation.

This entire study based on a vigorous work. All supervisors, librarians (especially the 24/7 Seaborne and Riverside Library), classmates and associated persons of this respected British institution; have lent their helping hands in this venture and without them, this systematic review could not be accomplished appropriately.

By this systematic review, I have got the advantage to work on this project with our Program Leader Pauline Alexander and had got opportunities to learn from her. Through her high supports, feedbacks and her excellent methods of teaching in everysteps, I think I can come up with a comprehensible systematic review.

Also, I express on record, my sense of gratitude and sincere thanks to all of them who have provided me all the necessary facilities, valuable guidance, information, encouragement, appreciation. There may be short comings, factual errors, a mistaken opinion which is all mine and I am alone responsible for those, but I will try for a better quality of writing in my future studies.

I would like to thank my teachers, parents, siblings, well-wishers, last but not the least, 'The One and Only Almighty'.
Thank you and Best wishes to all.....
Tarannum Rahman

DEDICATION

I dedicate this Systematic Review to the Almighty, my parents, teachers and well-wishers; who have guided me and supported me with patience and encouraged me to develop a better career in future life.

List of Abbreviations

Terms	Abbreviations
RCTs	Randomized Control Trials
ESRC	Economic and Social Research Council
RCN	The Royal College of Nursing
UoC	University of Chester
IT	Information Technology
W.H.O	World Health Organization
MRI	Magnetic Resonance Imaging
QALY	Quality Adjusted Life Years
DALY	Disability Adjusted Life Years

Keywords

Randomized Control Trials (RCTs), Dementia, Cognitive, Behavioural Therapy, Psychological Symptoms,Music Therapy, Clinical Trials;Quality of Life; Treatment Outcomes; Single-Blind Studies;Nursing Home Patients;REVMAN Analysis; Aged, 80 and Over; Aged; Male; Female; Geriatric Depression Scale; Questionnaires; ClinicalAssessment Tools; Psychological Tests; Scales; Interview Guides

Summary/ Abstract

The background of this study is to determine whether there is an association between music intervention and cognitive, behavioural and psychological effect in healthy older adults, and if so, music therapy intervention can be used as first-line non-pharmacological treatment. This study is a systematic review and meta-analysis of clinical trials that will examined the effects of music intervention. A comprehensive and systematic literature review was performed on PubMed, PscyhInfo, CINAHL, the Cochrane Library. A total of 31 studies were found relevant to the topics; all of them had an acceptable quality based on the CASP scale score. There was positive evidence to support the use of music intervention on treatment of cognitive,behavioural and psychological function of dementia patients in elderly.

The Music Therapy Checklist is useful for music therapists to monitor and evaluate the music therapeutic process. A list of different types of behaviorswere selected based on results derived from applying the Music Therapy Coding Scheme. The use of a checklist to code the events with a recording method based on 1-min. intervalsallows observation without data-processing systems and drastically reduces coding time. At the same time, the checklist tags the main factors in musical interaction.

Muñiz, R., Olazarán, J., Poveda, S., Lago, P., & Peña-Casanova, J. (2011). NPT-ES: A measure of the experience of people with dementia during non-pharmacological interventions. *Non-Pharmacological Therapies in Dementia*, 1(3), 1-11.

Raglio, A., & Gianelli, M. V. (2013). Music and music therapy in the management of behavioral disorders in dementia.

Raglio, A., et al. (2007). "Comparison of the Music Therapy Coding Scheme with the Music Therapy Checklist." Psychological Reports101(3): 875-880.

1994 by the American Academy of Neurology:

doi: http://dx.doi.org/10.1212/WNL.44.12.2308 *Neurology December 1994 vol. 44 no. 12* 2308

http://www.neurology.org/content/44/12/2308

We developed a new instrument, the Neuropsychiatric Inventory (NPI), to assess 10 behavioral disturbances occurring in dementia patients: delusions, hallucinations, dysphoria, anxiety, agitation/aggression, euphoria, disinhibition, irritability/lability, apathy, and aberrant motor activity. The NPI uses a screening strategy to minimize administration time, examining and scoring only those behavioral domains with positive responses to screening questions. Both the frequency and the severity of each behavior are determined. Information for the NPI is obtained from a caregiver familiar with the patient's behavior. Studies reported here demonstrate the content and concurrent validity as well as between-rater, test-retest, and internal consistency reliability; the instrument is both valid and reliable. The NPI has the advantages of evaluating a wider range of psychopathology than existing instruments, soliciting information that may distinguish among different etiologies of dementia, differentiating between severity and frequency of behavioral changes, and minimizing administration time.

A SYSTEMATIC REVIEW OF COGNITIVEANDBEHAVIOURALEFFECT OF MUSIC THERAPY ON OLDER ADULTS WITH DEMENTIA

1. INTRODUCTION

47.5 million people are affected with age-related neuro-cognitive andbehavioural disorder named as Dementia, and 1.9 million people have died due to this disease according to the world health report of 2015 whereas 7.7 million new cases are occurring every year (Candy, 2015). One in four people aged 85 and over; will have different forms of dementia; by the end of the year 2050 (HSCIC, 2016). However, in the year of 2013, this fatal psychological disease lead to 1.7 million annual deaths, whereas in 1990; there were only 0.8 million deaths per annum due to dementia; which indicates that the rate of affected patients and case fatality rate are increasing gradually (Konno, Kang &Makimoto, 2014).

Music therapy is a quick form of non-pharmacological, non-invasive intervention for the rising number of demented patients besides the medical as well as pharmacological intervention. Because these traditional interventions have proven their ineffectiveness and handled to side effects of medicinein demented patients (Vasionye& Madison, 2013).

Nationwide, about 10% of the population, develop dementia at some point in their lives. It is a common form of brain defects which occur due to theageing process and genetic abnormalities. Approximately half ofthe entire dementic population is over 85 years old and over. 3% individuals aged between 65–74 years have dementia in 2016; whereas 19% people with this disease aged between 75 - 84 years,which indicates that the percentage of individuals who are getting dementia is proportionate to the gradual increase of their age (Brett, Traynor&Stapley, 2016).

By the blessings of modern medicine where more people are living longer, dementia is becoming more and more common in the population which overrides the percentage ofcardiac illness, hypertension and other neurological age-related problems. Furthermore, for individuals with a younger age group, dementia is less frequent in the developing countries. Due to decrease risk factors and caring environment for the elderly persons, more carer within the family, family values and morals; dementia has not taken ittolls in countries like Bangladesh.Dementia isan excellentcause of disability among the old in various parts of the world. This fatal disease has increased the economic burden by which costs of care increases byUSD 604 billion a year worldwide in 2010. People with dementia are often physically and mentally restrained from a higher degree of benefit out of medication and pharmacological care which is necessary for their existence. Furthermore, theseelderly people could be an excellent source of knowledge, experience, wisdom for their future generations, but due to lack of self-consciousness, behavioural fluctuation, cognitive un-equilibrium, and so on; they are becoming the burden of the so-called societal aspect. Social stigma against these affected people is common because patients are not usually aware of their rights as well.

At present, for an example of dementia in the developed world, 8.5 million people are suffering from this fatal psychological illness out of 65.5 million total population in the United Kingdom; which is 1.3 % has been estimated to rise above another one million by the year 2021 stated by the Mapping Dementia Services In The South West Finland the Alzheimer's Society UK Report, 2017.

On the contrary, in developing countrieslike Bangladesh; it is estimated that people with dementia in Bangladesh will rise to 8,34,000 in 2030 and 21,93,000 in 2050 respectively.

Demented patientsin Bangladesh also have a growing concern related to increased social burden and challenges regarding thecost associated with dementia epidemic. For Bangladesh, bearing the world's eighth-largest population which is 164.8 million in 2017, patients with dementia are counted as 4.6 people million in 2017, which are 0.3% of thetotal population of Bangladesh. This comparision between developed and developing countries indicate that developed countries' older persons are more prone to get dementia than

8

developing countries population because of the social structure, race, religion, population density, morality, genetic factors, etc(Alzheimer's Society Bangladesh Report, 2017).

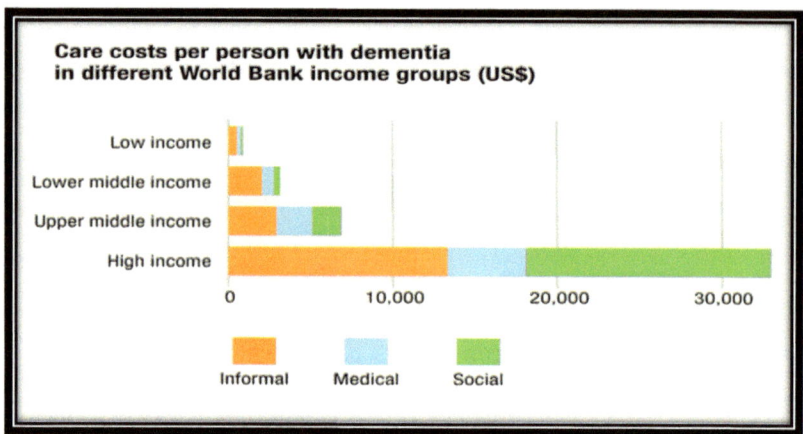

Figure 1: Alzheimer's Society, 2017

The costs of caring for these populations have been estimated currently to be around USD 8 billion for direct medical care, rising to over USD 20 billion if full communal costs are taken into contemplation, which is more than the combined costs of cancer and heart disease care. The majority of these expenses are for long-term residential care (40% of total expenditure) and informal caregivers (55% of total spending), with only 5% of costs going in primary and secondary care due to medication. Meanwhile the prevalence of dementia increases abruptly with time and person's age; these costs are set to escalate sharply in future due to the growth of the ageing population stated by a PhD Project Proposal named living well with dementia (Sung, Lee, & Watson, 2012).

DESCRIPTION OF THE CONDITION

Dementia is a neurological syndrome which consists of deterioration in memory, thinking and behaviour which leads to loss of ability to perform everyday activities. There are four common subtypes of dementia regarding the frequency of occurring disease and illness prevalence. Alzheimer's disease is the common type of dementia which comprises of 60–70% of total dementia patients according to WHO Report, 2016. Lewy-body- dementia (15%), vascular type of dementia(25%) andfrontotemporaldementia (3%) are the additional varieties of dementia. Less common causes include normal pressure hydrocephalus, Parkinson's disease, syphilis, and Creutzfeldt–Jakob disease among others (Van de Winkel, Fey, De Weerdt& Dom, 2004).

Beyond one category of dementia may occur in the same person in the same time. A small proportion of dementia cases are inherited in families. Dementia is reclassified under the neurocognitive disorder, with various components of severity. Diagnosis is usually based on the history of the illness, cognitive testing with medical imaging, blood testing used to rule out other possible causes, genetic or family history, etc. The mini-mental state examination is one commonly used cognitive test to assess the level of this disease. Efforts to prevent dementia include trying to decrease risk factors related to high blood pressure, stroke and other associated neurological illness.

The music therapy intervention is helpful in the state of stimulating the neuron cells by sound waves which will help the older adults to recover their previous degenerating neurons (Standring, 2015). Dementia is a broader type of brain disease that causes a long-term and often gradual decrease in the ability to think and remember; that is significant enough to affect a person's daily functioning. Other common symptoms include emotional and language problems and low motivation. A person's consciousness is usually not affected. Naturally, genetic, environmental and other associated conditions may cause dementia. A dementia diagnosis requires a change from a person's normal mental functioning and a greater decline than ageing. This disease also has a significant effect on the patient's family members, close relatives and caregivers.

Table 1: Diagnostic criteria for dementia

Type of dementia	Diagnostic criteria
Alzheimer's disease	Preferred criteria: NINCDS/ADRDA. Alternatives include ICD-10 and DSM-IV
Vascular dementia	Preferred criteria: NINDS-AIREN. Alternatives include ICD-10 and DSM-IV
Dementia with Lewy bodies	International Consensus criteria for dementia with Lewy bodies
Frontotemporal dementia	Lund-Manchester criteria, NINDS criteria for frontotemporal dementia
DSM-IV, Diagnostic and Statistical Manual of Mental Disorders, fourth edition; ICD-10, International Classification of Diseases, 10th revision; NINCDS/ADRDA, National Institute of Neurological and Communicative Diseases and Stroke/Alzheimer's Disease and Related Disorders Association; NINDS–AIREN, Neuroepidemiology Branch of the National Institute of Neurological Disorders and Stroke–Association Internationale pour la Recherche et l'Enseignement en Neurosciences.	

Figure 2: NICE Guideline and quality standard for dementia

DESCRIPTION OF INTERVENTION

The use of music therapy in older adults with dementia helps to stimulate communication and memory skills which have been reported by The Rebecca Centre for Music Therapy in New York, 2016. The Founder of the centre, John Carpenter and other licensed board-certified music therapists proved by their studies that listening to previously acquainted music and being involved in live music assist in making experiences come to life and empowers clients to get back into real life from the isolation which is superimposed by dementia(Sung, Lee, & Watson, 2012).However, the advantages of music therapy are theability to remember or gain the previous memories, positive changes in moods, attitudes towards life, emotional and psychological improvement of themind, a sense of control over life. It is a non-invasive procedure and non-meditational, but rather effective (Standring, 2015).

Music therapy is a non-pharmacological medication for pain, disability and discomfort according to the Age UK Report, (2016). According to WHO, 2016; some registered music therapist of USA, this therapy is used to maintain and increase levels of physical, psychological, social, and emotional functioning. Music is used as a sensory and intellectual stimulation which can help dementia patients to maintain and improve their quality of life (QOL), quality adjusted life years(QALY), etc.

Neuroscientists, now equipped with brain scanning technology, e.g. MRI, CT scan, PET CT(APPENDIX:4, FIGURE:6). Have a changed interest in finding how music affects our neural circuits.

How might the intervention work?

According to 'Dementia: Music and the Mind Report', May 2016; researchers in Finland using MRI, it was found that listening to music recruits not only the auditory areas (e.g. amygdala, fifth auditory nerves' pathways) of the brain but also employs large-scale neural networks. For instance, they discovered that the processing of musical or rhythmic impulse recruits motor areas by redirecting their pathways in the brain. It supports the idea that music and memory are closely interconnected. Limbic and gyrus areas of the brain, known to be associated with psychological and behavioural pathways which were found to be involved in rhythm. Processing of timbre and tonality, music is strongly associated with activation of the default memory pathways (Gray's Anatomy, 2014).

There is no cure for dementia, medications only reduce the symptoms.Cholinesterase inhibitors such as donepezil are often used and may be beneficial in mild to moderate disorder.However,theoverall benefit is very minor. Cognitive and behavioural interventions may be appropriate to improve the quality of life of people with dementia and their family members as well as caregivers. Educating and providing emotional support to the caregivers is also important.Exercise programs may be beneficial concerning activities of daily living and potentially improve outcomes. Treatment of behaviouralproblemswith antipsychotics is common but not usually recommended due to the little benefit and side effects, including an increased risk of death.

According to Vink et al., 2014; maintenance of the treatment often decreases due to carelessness of the family members, lack of knowledge of the practitioners, by WHO, 2016 (Wittwer, Webster, & Hill, 2013).

JUSTIFICATION

It is a global health problem which is increasing throughout the years, e.g. by the year 2030 the incidence of dementia people will be double, and by 2050 it will be triple according to WHO Report, 2016.

At present, 35.6 million people are living with dementia which is not only affecting them but also affecting family life, socioeconomic and health dimensions by increasing disability adjusted life years or DALY (Dr Margaret Chan, WHO Report, 2016)

Dementia is the principal reason of dependence and disability in the elderly person worldwide.the Framingham Heart Study assessed the temporal regoin damage in the incidence of dementia over last three decades which shows that it is increasing the average life expectancy of a human being so that economic burden will be increased exponentially as well (Satizabal, Beiser, Chouraki, Chêne, Dufouil, & Seshadri, 2016). This catastrophic cost destroys the economic stability of many poor households (WHO, 2016).

This non-communicable disease is one of the biggest challenges for the development of 21st Century (Mental Health Gap Action Program, 2008, High-level Meeting of United Nations General Assembly, 2011).

The overall estimated global expenditures of dementia were 604 billion US dollar in 2010. In high-income countries, informal nursing care and support cost 45%, and formal social care costs 40% of the majority of costs among all other medical expenses, which is 15% lower in low-income and lower-middle-income countries. Their social care and informal care cost are lesser because it is provided by their own family on an unpaid basis towards elderly as a cultural norm (WHO Report, 2016).

Cognitive, behavioural and psychological effects of music therapy on older adults with dementia were done in different settings in various occasions even with gold standard randomised control trials, case-control and cohort studies,and so forth(Raglio, 2015). However, itis not doneonmany occasions as a systematic review and meta-analysis. To fulfil this gap between studies, a systematic considerationof both qualitative and quantitative research in this related field will provide newer and precise stronger results and findings.

The use of music therapy in older adults with dementia helps to stimulate communication and memory skills which have been reported by The World famous and legendary Rebecca Centre for Music Therapy in New York, 2016. The Founder of the centre, John Carpenter and other licensed board-certified music therapist proved by their studies that listening to previously acquainted music and being involved in live music-making experiences come to life and empowers clients to get back into real life from the isolation which issuperimposed by dementia(Sung, Lee, & Watson, 2012).

However, the advantages of music therapy are the ability to remember or gain the previous memories, positive changes in moods, attitudes towards life, emotional and psychological improvement of the mind, a sense of control over life,etc. It is a non-invasive procedure and non-meditational, but rathereffective (Standring,2015).

Music therapy is anon-pharmacological medication for pain, disability and discomfortaccording to the Age UK Report, (2016). According to some registered music therapist of USA, this therapy is used to maintain or increase levels of physical,cognitive, behavioural, psychological, social, and emotional functioning. Music used as a sensory and intellectual stimulation can help which can sustain and improve quality of life (QALY) byMurfield et al.,2011.

For centuries, music has been known to tranquillise people without medication and withdraw the stress and tension by producing soothing sound waves. Neuroscientists, now equipped with brain scanning technology, e.g. MRI, CT scan, PET CT(APPENDIX:4, FIGURE:6), etc. have a changed interest in finding how music affects our neural circuits (Johnson, Deatrick&Oriel, 2012).

It is a global health problem which is increasing throughout the years e.g. by the year 2030 the incidence of dementia people will be double and by 2050 it will be triple according to WHO Report, 2016.

At present 35.6 million people are living with dementia which is not only affecting them but also affecting family life, socio-economic and health dimensions by increasing DALY (Dr. Margaret Chan, WHO Report, 2016)

Dementia is the principal reason of dependence and disability in the elderly person worldwide., The Framingham Heart Study assessed the temporal trends in the incidence of dementia over last three decades which shows that it is increasing with the average life expectancy of human being so economic burden will be increased exponentially as well (Satizabal, Beiser, Chouraki, Chêne, Dufouil, &Seshadri, 2016). This catastrophic cost destroys the economic stability of many poor household (WHO, 2016).

This non-communicable disease is one of the major challenges for the development of 21st Century (Mental Health Gap Action Program, 2008, High level Meeting of United Nations General Assembly, 2011)

The overall estimated global expenditures of dementia were 604 billion US dollar in 2010. In high-income countries, informal nursing care and support cost 45% and formal social care costs 40% of the majority of costs among all other medical costs, which is 15% lower in low-income and lower-middle-income countries. Their social care and informal care cost are lesser because it is provided by their own family in an unpaid basis towards elderly as a cultural norm (WHO Report, 2016).

Cognitive, behavioural and psychological effects of music therapy on older adults with dementia were done in different settings in various occasions even with gold standard randomized control trials, case-control and cohort studies, etc.(Raglio, 2015). But it is not done in any occasions as a systematic review and/or meta-analysis. To fulfil this gaps between studies, a systematic review with both qualitative and quantitative studies in this related field will provide newer and precise stronger results and findings.

The use of music therapy in older adults with dementia helps to stimulate communication and memory skills which has been reported by World famous and legendary Rebecca Center for Music Therapy in New York, 2016. The Founder of the centre, John Carpenter and other licensed board certified music therapist proved by their studies that listening to previously acquainted music and being involved in live music make experiences come to life and empowers clients to get back into real life from the isolation which is superimposed by dementia(Sung, Lee, & Watson, 2012).However, the advantages of music therapy are ability to remember or gain the previous memories, affirmative changes in moods, attitudes towards life, emotional and psychological improvement of mind, a sense of control over life,etc. It is a non-invasive procedure and non-meditational, but rathereffective (Standring ,2015).

Music therapy is anon-pharmacological medication for pain, disability and discomfortaccording to the Age UK Report, (2016). According to some registered music therapist of USA, this therapy is used to maintain or increase levels of physical, psychological, social, and emotional functioning. Music used as a sensory and intellectual stimulation can help maintain and improve quality of life (QALY).

For centuries, music has been known to tranquilize people without medication and withdraw the stress and tension by producing soothing sound waves.

Neuroscientists, now equipped with brain scanning technology e.g. MRI, CT scan, PET CT(APPENDIX:4, FIGURE:6), etc. have a changed interest in finding how music affects our neural circuits.

According to 'Dementia: Music and the Mind Report', May, 2016; researchers in Finland using MRI, it was found that listening to music recruits not only the auditory areas (e.g. amygdala, 5th auditory nerves' pathways) of the brain, but also employs large-scale neural networks. For instance, they discovered that the processing of musical or rhythmic impulserecruits motor areas by redirecting their pathways in the brain. It supports the idea that music and memory are closely interconnected. Limbic and gyrus areas of the brain, known to be associated with psychological and behavioural pathways which were found to be involved in rhythm. Processing of timbre and tonality, music is strongly associated with activations of the default memory pathways (Gray's Anatomy, 2014).

WHY IS IT IMPORTANT TO DO THIS REVIEW?

According to 'Dementia: Music and the Mind Report', May 2016; researchers in Finland using MRI, it was found that listening to music recruits not only the auditory areas (e.g. amygdala, fifth auditory nerves' pathways) of the brain but also employs large-scale neural networks. For instance, the scientists discovered that the processing of musical or rhythmic impulse recruits motor areas by redirecting their pathways in the brain. It supports the idea that music and memory are closely interconnected. Limbic and gyrus areas of the brain, known to be associated with psychological and behavioural pathways which were found to be involved in rhythm. Processing of tonality, music or sound waves are strongly associated with activation of the default memory pathways (Gray's Anatomy, 2014).

Table 2 Effectiveness of different types of music interventions (Vasionye& Madison, 2013)

Characteristic of intervention	Sample Size (number of studies)	Mean ES	CI (95%)	Q (a = 0.05)
Listening	250 (10)	1.61*	1.25; 1.96	76.79
Active music therapy	188 (8)	0.44	-0.09; 0.97	0.54†

Recorded music	250 (10)	1.61*	1.25; 1.96	76.80
Live music	132 (6)	0.54	-0.08; 1.16	0.03†
Group intervention	320 (12)	2.09*	1.54;2.64	52.15
Individual intervention	118 (6)	1.00*	0.48;1.53	8.62†
Selected music	233 (9)	1.38*	1.07; 1.70	84.07
Individualised music	135 (7)	0.71	-0.43; 1.85	0.48†
Classical/ relaxation music	135 (5)	1.66*	1.30; 2.02	74.92
Popular/native music	126 (4)	0.54	-0.56; 1.64	0.05†

*Effect size (ES) is statistically significant.

†Q non-significant, ES homogeneous.

Why an empirical research is not carrying out here; instead of a systematic review?

Systematic reviews are the gold standard of all the research methodologies. They are transparent, lack of biases, cannot be replicated (Boland, Cherry and Dickson, 2014). In the study of Bergenholtz&Kvist, 2014; identified intervention 'music therapy in dementia patient' will be investigated and addressed by this research by carrying out a rigorous data analysis; which is not done in empirical studies. These evidence-based findings of the systematic review can be used to formanew intervention for ademntia patient, which also navigates towards a well-developed empirical study. It also prepares the groundwork for thedevelopment of clinical guidelines and assistsdementia caregivers in decision-making to choose wise intervention(Higgins & Green, 2011).

2. LITERATURE REVIEW

Epidemiology of dementia

Prevalence and impact:

The term 'Dementia' had been stated in different ways in different articles, journals and books. Cognative, behavioural and psychological symptoms of dementia (BPSDs) have a melodramatic effect on persons with dementia (PWD), especially in the progressive stages of the disease. Non-pharmacological management, comprising with music interventions, have been proposed for the reduction of BPSDs in PWDs (Shagam, 2009).The number of people with dementia are on the rise dramatically with increased longevity. The core dementia symptoms are cognitive, behavioural and psychological deterioration mainly. In case of doing literature review, the selected studies/papers are written in English language, studies evaluating the psychological, behavioural, cognitive function before and after music therapy intervention to manage symptoms of dementia patients, studies with a comparator groups, separate groups or before/after comparisons, studies with quantitative results in which all participants had dementia in different levels and various types. Types and levels of dementia had not been separated in the criteria of the studies so in most of the studies calculated the effect size (ES) rather than meta-analysis because of various variables. The most widely used and recommended (Jeon et al., 2011) clinical tool for evaluating BPSD is the Neuropsychiatric Inventory (NPI) (Cummings et al., 1994) and for cognitive evaluation most of the studies done MMSE (Mini-Mental State Examination/Score) since 1973, discovered by Paul. MMSE is essential in quantitative assessment of cognitive performance with high reliability and validity. There are five types of dementia: Alzheimer's disease, Vascular dementia, frontotemporal dementia, dementia with Lewy bodies, Young onset dementia. Alzheimer's disease(prevalence 60-70%) cause poor memory function, cognitive disability, poor insight, lack of awareness and language dysfunction. It develops gradually from mild to severe form including disorientation which hampers their everyday performance.Vascular dementia or multi-infarct dementia (MID), is the second most common type of dementia, which is a most

21

common after effect of strokes. As a result, it causes gradual deterioration of memory following slow recovery period, but language and communication are not affected in this case of dementia patients. On the other hand, frontotemporal dementia or pic'd disease affect behaviour and personality which can be found in younger people aged between 45-65 years old, but this type of dementia can be confused with depression, psychosis or OCD (obsessive compulsive disorder) as dementia is not common in younger people, though there is Young Onset Dementia which is unexpected as well. Dementia with Lewy bodies, cognitive impairment can fluctuate, and movements are particularly affected, with poor motor control. Tremors may be noticed in Parkinson's disease. Due to the nerve cell damage of Lewy bodies, hallucinations are often present in those with this type of dementia. These hallucinations can be both visual and auditory. Memory is often less affected. As with all dementias, Lewy bodies are progressive, and symptoms will worsen over time.

Introduction

In the beginning, I would like to focus on the concept of dementia and its various treatments that are needed to care for the older adults in the community properly. Various researchers discuss on the cognitive theory, behavioural theory, physiological approach and the benefit of the music therapy for the treatment of dementia in the context of older adults. The variables will be discussed critically based on the past studies and the secondary research studies. In this section, the selected research issues have concluded, and it has discussed how the older adult patients with dementia are treated by the health and social care organisations through the newer approach of Music Therapy.

Past studies

From the previous studies over the dementia issues biologically, it has expressed that the issue dementia has been prevalent in the age of people over the age of 65 years. Kanatli et al., (2007) stated that about 10% of the people who are over the age of 65 years had faced this issue of dementia and 47% of the people are at the age of 85 years are suffering from this issue. From the announcement, it has expressed that ageing is a universal issue. As a result,

22

the brain alters due to such physical and mental changes that include 'apoptosis, oxidative stress, telomere loss, neuroendocrine alterations, autoimmune changes, and others' are affecting the mental ability of the human being by Theories Of Aging And Dementia- Alzbrain (n.d.). The World Health Organization (2012) added to the theory that worldwide more than 47 million people are facing the issue of dementia and among them, most of the patients are in their older age. From the statement, it can be explicited clearly that the issue of dementia is seen mostly among the older adults. The cognitive functions are improved by using music therapy which has been implemented by the healthcare organisations for treating these patients. From the past studies, it has concluded that for dementia, music therapy is the standard issue that has proved its effectiveness over standard care through different randomised control trials (RCTs) in older adults.

Concept of Dementia with older adults

The issue dementia is the typical issue that affects people most after a specific age group because, by the age, the mental ability reduces, and hence a person becomes unable to remember numerous things. Prince et al., (2016) mentioned in the research paper that after the specific age group, 65 and above, the nervous system of a human being become weaker that causes the person unable to remember anything for a long time. The report of WHO has interpreted that from a long time the issue of dementia has seen in the community because it is not a disease, it is an effect of the natural cause named ageing. WHO has also presented a fact in the report that the patients of dementia are rising every year. Almost 47 million of people worldwide are facing the issue of dementia that is expected to reach nearly 131 million by the year of 2050 (World Health Organization, 2012).

Impact of music therapy on cognitive functions of older adult patients with dementia

The cognitive theory is being used by the health and social care organisations in the community for taking care of dementia older adults. Mac Pherson et al., (2002) specified that the issue of dementia is the part of a human age that is affecting the mental ability of the human being after a specific age group of 65 and above. Vink et al., (2014) added that the cognitive theory is one of the best as well as the most effective techniques that are helpful for taking care of the old adults, suffering from dementia. The statement has presumed that a health and social care organisation might follow cognitive function assessment in the community such as mapping of dementia, self-assessment chart and small comprehensions at the workplace. Johnson et al., (2012) added to the discussion that, people who have dementia are not an actual patient, only the difference is their mental capability reduces, cognative function deteriotes with their age.The statement has deduced that the dementia patients need a universal care from the health service provider.

Impact of music therapy on behavioural and psychological functions of older adult patients with dementia

The behavioural and the psychological functions or activities increases after the music therapy performed by the healthcare service providers which are the fundamental factor that put an impact on the mind of the dementia patients. In the above therapy, the cognitive, behavioural and psychological functions have been enhanced with the mean for taking care of the dementia patients. Wortmann (2012) explained that, in the workplace, there should be a mutual understanding between the behavioural approach of the service provider with the patient while providing them with music therapy. The statement has perceived that it might be possible that the patient of dementia failed to understand the behavioural approach of the service provider. Hence, it is the responsibility of the service provider or the music therapist that he should understand the behaviour and help the patient.

Benefits of music therapy on the older adults with dementia

From the research paper of Raglio et al., (2015), it has been observed that the people who are suffering from the issue of dementia in the community love to listen to music. From the research paper of Fanget al.,(2017), it has even interpreted that the music therapy acted positively at the workplace for entertaining the dementia patient as well as treating them and helping them recover and activate previous memory. In favour of this statement, it has been concluded that music has a rhythm that attracts the patients as well as increase the frequency level of the mind. Further, this helps the service provider to control the mind as well as the behaviour of the patient. The statement has even deduced that the wave of the music psychologically connects the mind of the patient with the rhythm that further helps the service provider to take care of that patient. From the discussion, it has been concluded that the music therapy is a compelling factor as well as a beneficial factor that helps a dementia patient to remember any information quickly.

3. METHODOLOGY

Methods are the technique to gather data and analyse it and methodology is the process of doing the research which is a design lying behind the choice and use of methods (Parahoo, 2006).This study has been done by following the nine steps of doing a systematic review (Boland, 2012) using quantitative research approach: writing a systematic review research proposal (step 1), literature review(step 2), screening for research relevant titles and abstracts(step 3), obtaining papers (step 4), and full text (step 5),quality assessment (step 6), data extraction (step7),analysis and synthesis (step8), writing up and editing the whole systematic review (step 9) by Boland et al., 2014. A systematic review is a gold standard way to do secondary research which locates, evaluate and combine the best available evidence relating to specific studies. Here, the RCTs that are relevant to this study have been selected and analysed through meta-analysis (Gray, 2014).

Research paradigm (Beauchamp & Childress, 2008) is the theoretical and philosophical process of doing any research which has different approaches according to the research questions and criteria of research designs. It reflects the values, attitudes of the researchers which impinge the research design, data collection; here gathering all primary data from all the relevant randomised control trials, methods, nature of investigations involved in the field of study (Bowling, 2014).

In case of following research paradigm (Denscombe, 2007), this systematic review has followed positivist research approach, which is a process of quantifying social phenomena step by step; whereas regarding epistemology, it is objectivism.The systematic review has followed a deductive process of positivism which is emphasising and quantifying specific concepts, verifying researcher's gaps and hunches. It has fixed design according to the methodology section and seeks generalised approach while selecting RCTs. Internal and external validity and reliability have been kept in mind while selecting the RCTs (Pink, 2007). According to Punch, 2014; there is an alternative paradigm named as a naturalistic or interpretative paradigm, which has inductive, qualitative, flexible design, seeks pattern, not ageneralisation, just opposite to the positivism's paradise. There is also another combined form of research paradigm named as a mixed method which combines both the qualitative and quantitative research approaches in the systematic review. Here the quantitative approach has been chosen based on the research question and study selection criteria which are relevant to the topics of this study (ESRC,2012; Department of Health, 2005 & Office of Public Sector Information, 1998).

Here, in case of the research process, in the first step'epistemology', objectivism has been chosen; according to the theory of knowledge according to the lecture-3of Research Module and Crotty, 1998; the foundation of social studies. Here, experimental research designs, RCTs have been chosen as per methodology section and statistical measurement, the techniques used in the data gathering and analysing process. Furthermore, there is no pragmatic approach or core principles; described in Denscombe, 2007; for doing any systematic review. Based on the research questions, methods, as well as methodology, has been formed and shaped to do a review.

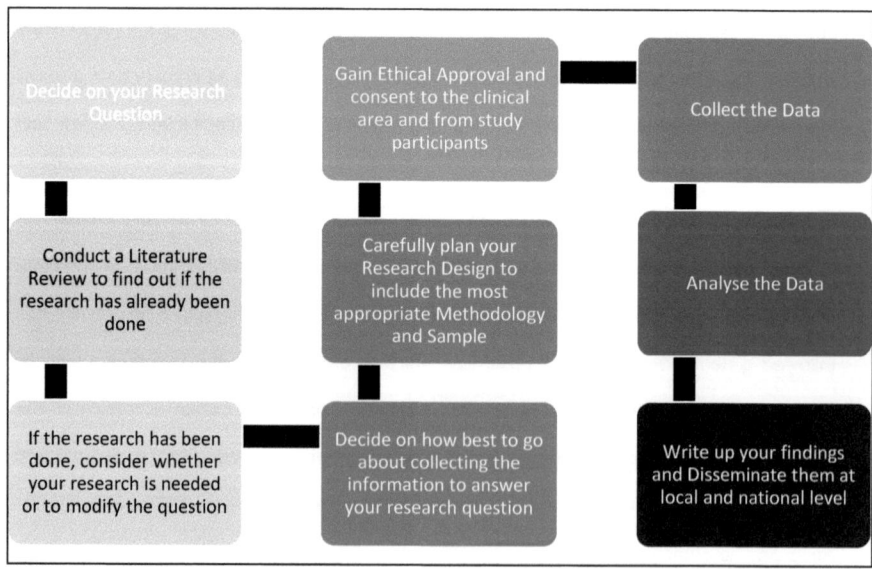

Figure 3: Research Process (Watson & Keady, 2008)

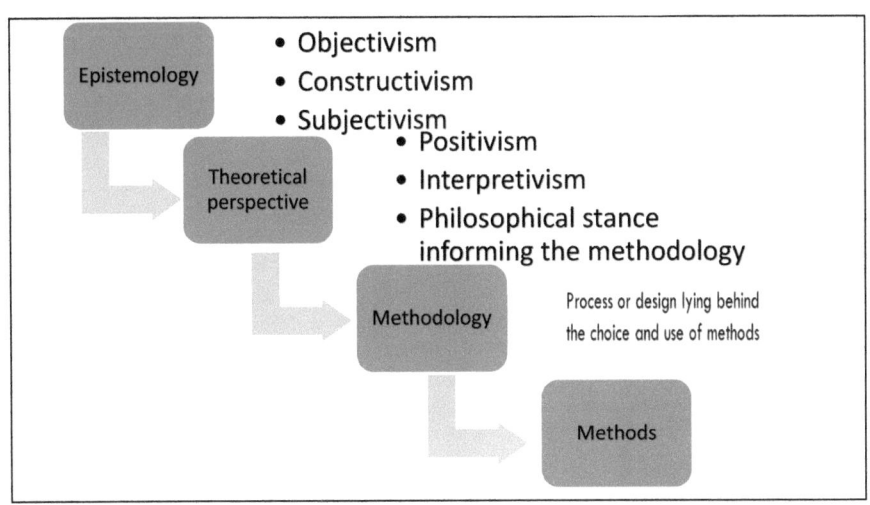

Figure 4 RESEARCH STAGES (Watson R & Keady (2008)

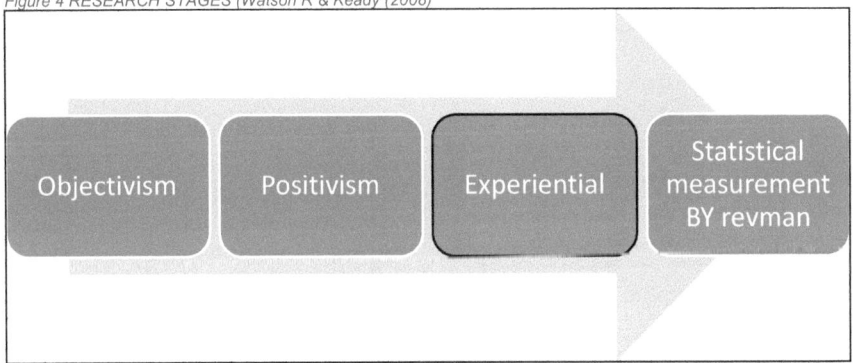

Figure 5: Research Steps (Followed) (Watson R & Keady (2008)

AUTHOR	TITLE	COUNTRY	AGE (RANGE)	SETTING	SAMPLE SIZE	SEVERITY/STAGE OF GE	INTERVENTION				OUTCOMES	RESULT
							Exp. music	Control intervention	Frequency & length	Provider		
Ridder et al., 2013	Individual music therapy for agitation in dementia: An exploratory RCT	Denmark & Norway	66-96	Nursing home	Exp (21) con(21)	MMSE:7.54 GDS:5.67	Individual MT	Standard Care	2times/ wk for 6wks	Music therapist	CMAI- frequency; CMAI: disruptiveness	Frequency of agitation decrease during MT whereas; increase during standard care

29

Effectiveness of group music intervention on agitated behaviour in elderly person with dementia	Taiwan	65-97 (82)	Aged care facility	Exp. 49 Con.51 MMSE:13.30 Moderate:62%	group music therapy	Usual care	Twice/wk for six wks	Research er got music therapy course	Chinese version: CMAI	Agitation significantly decreases
Lin et al., 2011										

30

Study										
Sung et al., 2012	A group music intervention using percussion instruments with familiar music to reduce anxiety and agitation of institutionalize dolder? >][< =o;pazadults with /dementiat/	Taiwan	80.4	residential care facility	Exp. 27 Con. Mild to moderate	group music therapy with familiar music	Usual care	Twice/wk for 6wks	Research assistant trained in music intervention	CMAI	The reduction of agitation between two groups was not significantly different, compared to control group

Sung et al., 2006	Taiwan	77.61	residential care facility	Exp. 18 Con. Moderate to severe	group music therapy with familiar music	Usual care	Twice/wk for six wks	Research assistant trained in music interventio n	CMAI-Modified	Agitation decreases in experimental group
The effects of group music with movement intervention agitated behaviours of institution-zed elders with dementia in Taiwan										

32

Cooke et al., 2010	An RCT exploring the effect of music on quality of life and depression in older people with dementia	Griffith university,	75-94	Care home	Exp (24) Con (23)	MMSE:16,51 mild-moderate	live familiar group music	Reading activity.	three times/wk for 8wks	musicians	CMAI-short form	MT did not decrease agitation

METHODS

Study selection criteria for doing literature review:

Included studies:

Jaded scales has been followed to select the studies from relevant randomized control trial in the field of music therapy on dementia patients and those studies have been chosen to do further systematic review in this area who have scored above three in the total score of five according to the lecture of 'Systematic Review' by Andy Mabhala and Ridley, (2012).

Those studies which show randomised control trials on dementia patients who are older adults and taking music therapies

No restriction was placed on the language or publication status of the papers.

Studies published between 1990 and 2006 were included. This date restriction was imposed to obtain data relevant to the current health and social care settings.

Excluded studies:

Dementia patient who is older adults taking other therapies rather than the music therapy in the studies

Dementia patient who is less than 60 to 85 years' old in the studies

Dementia patient who is 60 to 85 years old taking part in other studies rather than the randomised control trials

SEARCH STRATEGY:

Search Methods for the Identification of Literature Review:

More widely used electronic databases were selected for the search, including CINAHL, Pub Med, HINARI, Google Scholar and several websites. To identify articles for literature review, we combined four search themes using the Boolean operator "and", "or" &"nor"(Boland, Cherry and Dickson, 2014).

The search strategy up to Jan 15, 2017, identified 1385 titles and abstracts which include 64 in PubMed using (Dementia" AND "Music Therapy" AND "Randomized Control Trials"), 476 in CINAHL (Using Dementia" AND "Intervention" AND "Randomized Control Trials"), 18 in Cochrane Library, 23 in ProQuest, 11 in VecNet and other grey literature in several websites.

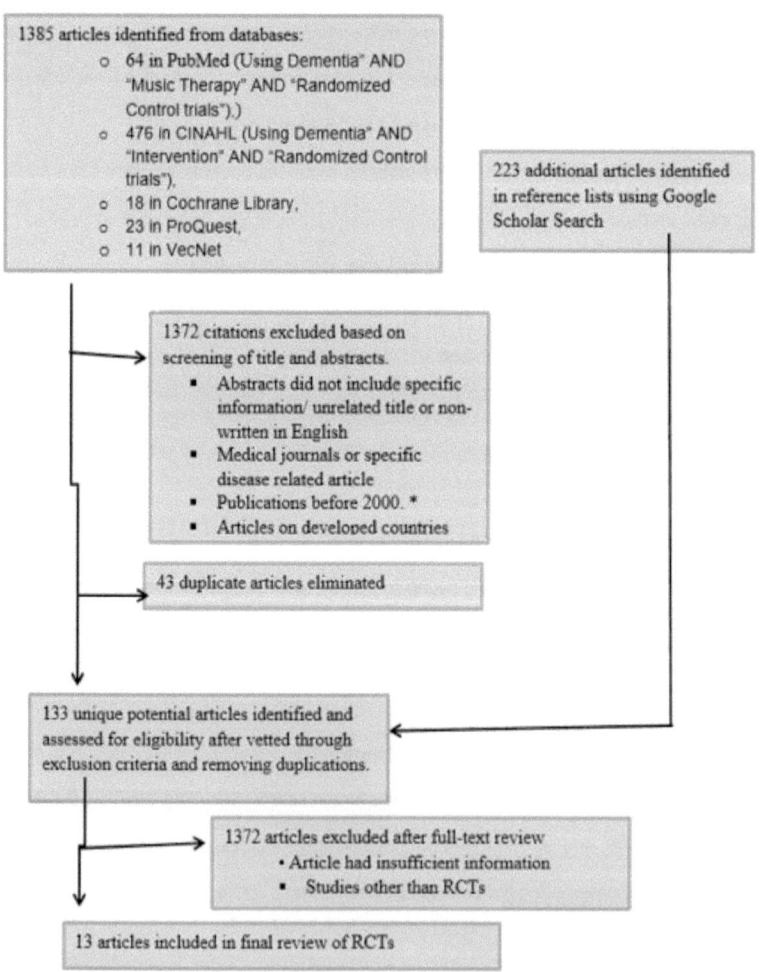

Conceptual Framework:

The inter relationshipbetween these factors of Aging and Health has been displayed by the theoretical framework and presented as Appendix 3.

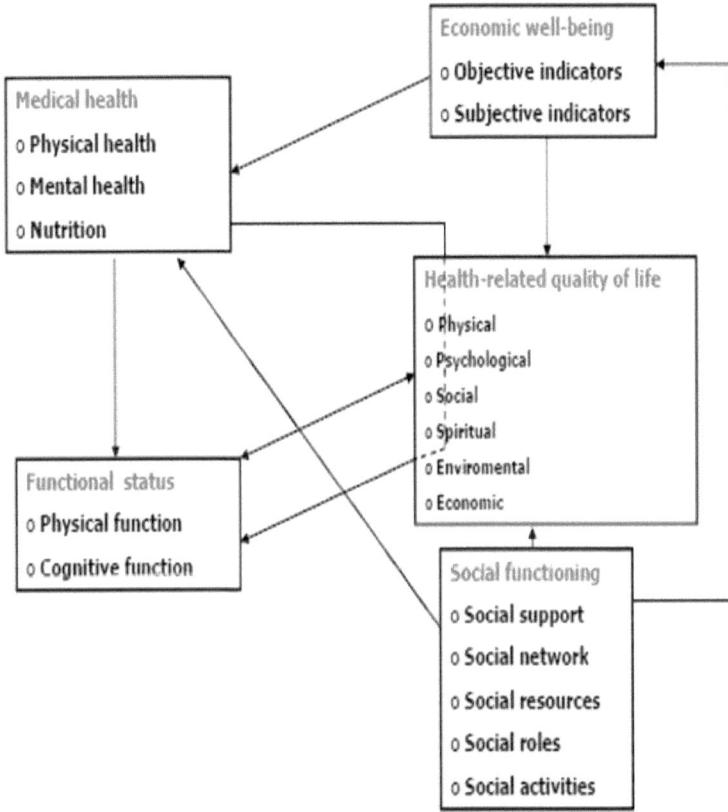

Aims and objectives

Research Aims: (Boland, Cherry and Dickson, 2014)

To measure/identify cognitive, behavioural and psychological effects of music therapy on older adults with dementia by this secondary study (systematic review) from previous primary studies (here primary studies are randomised control trials)

OBJECTIVES: (Boland, Cherry and Dickson, 2014)

General Objective:

To cognitive and behavioural effect of music therapy on older adults with dementia

Specific Objective:

The specific objectives of the proposed systematic review study:

To evaluate the effect of music therapy on cognitive functions of older adult patients with dementia

To assess the effect of music therapy on behavioural functions of older adult patients with dementia

To evaluate the effect of music therapy on psychological functions of older adult patients with dementia

To measure the benefit of music therapy in dementia patient

Research Questions :(Boland, Cherry and Dickson, 2014).

General Research Questions:

To cognitive and behavioural effect of music therapy on older adults with dementia

Specific Research Questions:

The specific objectives of the proposed systematic review study:

To evaluate the effect of music therapy on cognitive functions of older adult patients with dementia

To assess the effect of music therapy on behavioural functions of older adult patients with dementia

To evaluate the effect of music therapy on psychological functions of older adult patients with dementia

To measure the benefit of music therapy in dementia patient

Research Hypothesis:(Boland, Cherry and Dickson, 2014).

Null Hypothesis (H_0):

There is no association between improvement of cognitive and behavioural function of an older adult with dementia and receiving music therapy

Alternative Hypothesis (H₀):

There is association between improvement of cognitive and behavioural function of an older adult with dementia and receiving music therapy

METHODOLOGY OF THE REVIEW:(Boland, Cherry and Dickson, 2014):

Here, in this systematic review, positivist research paradigm has been followed which comprises of deductive process, emphasis on specific concepts, verification of researchers' hunches, fixed design, emphasis on measured, quantitative information; statistical analysis, generalisation (Crotty,1998).

Methods:

Study Type:

Systematic Reviewwith meta-analysis (Boland, Cherry, & Dickson, 2013&Ridley, 2012)

Type of Intervention:

Cognitive and Behavioral Therapy Especially Music Therapy in Dementia Patients (Boland, Cherry, & Dickson, 2013&Ridley, 2012).

Type of Outcome:

Regeneration of the neuron towards restore of memory to improve the condition of dementia (Boland, Cherry, & Dickson, 2013&Ridley, 2012)

Study/ Research Design/ selection of studies:

(Boland, Cherry, & Dickson, 2013&Ridley, 2012).

Randomized control trials (RCTs)

Systematic Review of related Randomized Control Trials (RCTs)

Randomized Control Trials (RCTs) with other additional studies, e.g. case-control, cohort studies, etc.

Study site:

Regardless of all RCTs settings (Boland, Cherry, & Dickson, 2013&Ridley, 2012)

Study population/Participants:

(Boland, Cherry, & Dickson, 2013&Ridley, 2012)

Adult aged between with 60 to 85 years old with dementia and receiving music therapy in the primary research of those randomised control trials

Eligibility Criteria:

(Boland, Cherry, & Dickson, 2013&Ridley, 2012).

Inclusion criteria:

Dementia patients who are older adults (60 to 85 years old) and taking music therapies in Randomized control trials (RCTs)(Boland, Cherry, & Dickson, 2013&Ridley, 2012).

Exclusion criteria:

Dementia patient who is less than 60 and more than 85 years' old

Dementia patient who is older adults taking other therapies than the music therapy

Dementia patient who is less than 60 to 85 years' old not participating inrandomised control trials (Boland, Cherry, & Dickson, 2013&Ridley, 2012).

Data Extraction and Management:

(Boland, Cherry, & Dickson, 2013&Ridley, 2012)

Quality assurance and critical appraisal of included studies have been shown in CASP Tools in APPENDIX:7.

Quality assurance:

(Boland, Cherry, & Dickson, 2013&Ridley, 2012)

For quality control, critical review of ethical approval will be done, and ethical approval form will be filled up and submitted after this proposal's acceptation by the authority. After obtaining the ethical approval from the department of Research of University of Chester according to the guidance of UoC, 2014, the systematic review will be started. Biases havebeen discussed in Appendix 11, table 5; according to Boland, Cherry, & Dickson, 2013&Ridley, 2012.

Randomized control trials based papers were selected only for doing the systematic review as we all know that Randomized control trials are the gold standard for all studies. However, within all studies, because of small sample size of these every Randomized control trials, the result is not as much as strong as a systematic review. For quality control of ethical issues, critical consideration of ethical issues and approval will be taken from the authority before starting the routinereview. CASP tool has been used to assure the quality control of the papers and critical appraisal of included studies. RCTs have been chosen by rating through Jaded scale for quality control of the journal: (Boland, Cherry, & Dickson, 2013&Ridley, 2012).

Data collection procedure/technique:

(Boland, Cherry, & Dickson, 2013&Ridley, 2012)

Gathering all randomised control trials from all available search engines, databases, e.g. Cochrane, CINAHL, PUBMED, etc. There are two type of data in this systematic review according the definition of systematic review i.e. primary data which had been taken previously in those selected thirteen randomized control trials and the secondary data which will be used from those randomized control trials to get a better and precise result (Boland, Cherry, & Dickson, 2013).

Data analysis:

(Boland, Cherry, & Dickson, 2013&Ridley, 2012)

Thematic analysis will be done for the qualitative part of the data either by the guideline of Miles Huberman's three stage analysis andDenscombe's five stage analysis (Boland, Cherry, & Dickson, 2013;Denscombe, 2007&Ridley, 2012). RevMan version 5.0 will be used for the quantitative data analysis to do the meta-analysis to evaluate all the RCT results

Data collection Method:

(Boland, Cherry, & Dickson, 2013&Ridley, 2012).

Obtaining all data from the randomised control trials, which are the primary studies for this systematic review and meta-analysis.

Study Period:

Tentatively seven months only (1stMarch 2017 to 30th Oct 2017) graphically presented in Appendix 8.

Validity and Reliability:

(Boland, Cherry, & Dickson, 2013&Ridley, 2012).

Music therapy (MT) has been proposed as valid and reliable approach to the evaluation of cognitive, behavioral and psychological symptoms (BPSD) and benefit ofmusic therapy (MT) in dementia according to Raglio, 2015 in the effect of Active Music Therapy and Individualized Listening to Music on Dementia: A Multicenter Randomized Controlled Trial'.CASP tool has been used to reassure all the points of internal and external validity, reliability and maintain the quality of both primary and secondary data of the papers and critical appraisal of included studies(Boland, Cherry, & Dickson, 2013&Ridley, 2012).

Ethical Consideration

(Boland, Cherry, & Dickson, 2013 & Ridley, 2012): Appendix 7

Ethical approval is obtained from the institutional review board, here the ethical review committee of the research department of the University of Chester. By the consent of Respected Supervisors, an ethical approval form was approved which was mentioning about the study objectives, procedures, benefits and risks of the study.

Six major ethical principles will be maintained throughout the period of research, i.e. beneficence (welfare of participants, to do good), non-malfeasance (to cause no harm), fidelity (the development of a trusting relationship between the researcher and participant), justice (being fair, veracity (truthfulness) and confidentiality (to maintain and protect information on the participant) (Beauchamp & Childress, 2008; Bowling, 2014; Denscombe, 2014; Punch, 2014).

Study or Subgroup	MT Mean [MMSE]	SD [MMSE]	Total	SC Mean [MMSE]	SD [MMSE]	Total	Weight	Mean Difference IV, Random, 95% CI [MMSE]
A Van de Winckel et al., 2004	16.93	3.66	27	16.39	3.9	23	38.4%	0.54 [-1.57, 2.65]
Ceccato et al., 2012	15.53	4.44	15	11	4	10	24.3%	4.53 [1.18, 7.88]
Lin et al, 2011	14.24	6.39	49	13.5	4.6	51	37.3%	0.74 [-1.45, 2.93]
Total (95% CI)			91			84	100.0%	1.58 [-0.52, 3.69]

Heterogeneity: Tau² = 1.85, Chi² = 4.33, df = 2 (P = 0.11); I² = 54%

Test for overall effect: Z = 1.47 (P = 0.14)

Risk of bias legend

(A) Random sequence generation (selection bias)

(B) Allocation concealment (selection bias)

(C) Blinding of participants and personnel (performance bias)

(D) Blinding of outcome assessment (detection bias)

(E) Incomplete outcome data (attrition bias)

(F) Selective reporting (reporting bias)

(G) Other bias

44

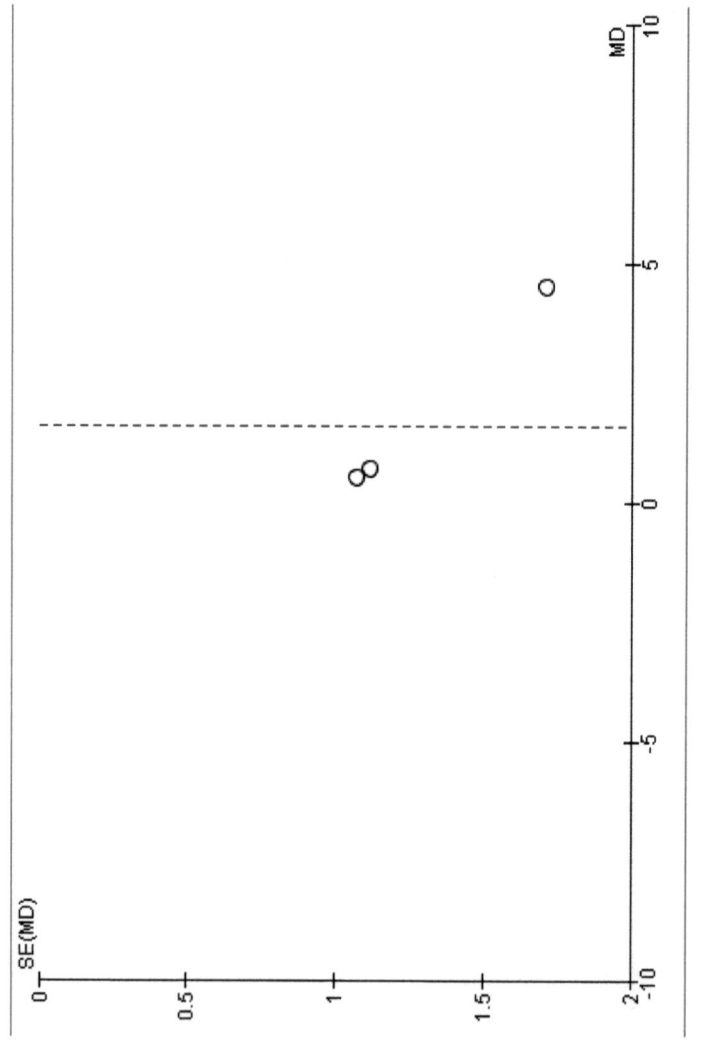

Study or Subgroup	music therapy Mean [CMAI]	SD [CMAI]	Total	standard care Mean [CMAI]	SD [CMAI]	Total	Weight	Mean Difference IV, Random, 95% CI [CMAI]
LIN et al, 2011	36.37	10.64	49	38.55	10.27	51	15.0%	-2.18 [-6.28, 1.92]
Ridder et al., 2013	26.09	13.54	17	28	18.15	19	3.0%	-1.91 [-12.30, 8.48]
Sung et al., 2006	3.44	1.29	18	4.5	1.64	18	49.9%	-1.06 [-2.02, -0.10]
Sung et al., 2012	32.7	4.98	27	51	2.96	28	32.1%	1.70 [-0.47, 3.87]
Total (95% CI)			**111**			**116**	**100.0%**	**-0.37 [-2.22, 1.48]**

Heterogeneity: Tau² = 1.54; Chi² = 5.76, df = 3 (P = 0.12); I² = 48%
Test for overall effect: Z = 0.39 (P = 0.70)

Standard Care   Music Therapy

Risk of bias legend
(A) Random sequence generation (selection bias)
(B) Allocation concealment (selection bias)
(C) Blinding of participants and personnel (performance bias)
(D) Blinding of outcome assessment (detection bias)
(E) Incomplete outcome data (attrition bias)
(F) Selective reporting (reporting bias)
(G) Other bias

46

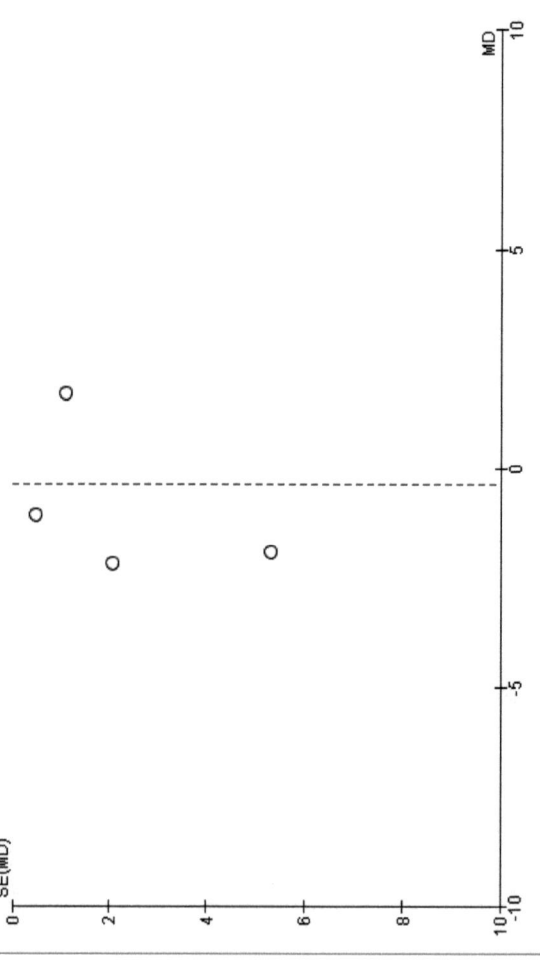

Reference List

Internal References:

Age UK Report, (2016). Retrieved on 19th Dec 2016 fromhttp://www.ageuk.org.uk/health-wellbeing/conditions-illnesses/dementia-and-music/

Alzheimer's SocietyUK Report, 2017. Retrieved on 19th Aug 2017fromhttps://www.alzheimers.org.uk/info/20091/what_we_think/93/demography

Alzheimer's Society BangladeshReport, 2017. Retrieved on 19th Aug 2017 fromhttp://alzheimerbd.com/dementia-statistics/

Beauchamp, T., Childress, J. (2008). *Principles of biomedical ethics*, 6th Ed, Oxford University Press: Oxford.

Boland, A., Cherry, M. G., & Dickson, R. (Eds.). (2013). *Doing a systematic review: A student's guide*. Sage. Retrievedon 19th Dec 2016 fromhttps://books.google.co.uk/books?hl=en&lr=&id=AO-GAwAAQBAJ&oi=fnd&pg=PP1&dq=boland+doing+a+systematic+review&ots=34xXE5h_Jf&sig=ofcJW3nUPhCDvpvqmyt2LZbofck#v=onepage&q=boland%20doing%20a%20systematic%20review&f=false

Bowling, A., (2014). Research methods in health, investigating health and health services, 4th Ed, Open University Press: Maidenhead

Brett, L., Traynor, V., & Stapley, P. (2016). Effects of Physical Exercise on Health and Well-Being of Individuals Living with a Dementia in Nursing Homes: A Systematic Review. *Journal of The American Medical Directors Association, 17*(2), 104-116. doi:10.1016 /j. jamda.2015.08.016

British Economic and Social Research Council (ESRC), (2012). *Framework for research ethics.* Retrieved on 19th Dec 2016 from http://www.esrc.ac.uk/about-esrc/information/research-ethics.aspx

Candy, M. (2015). The importance of innovation in care homes. *Nursing and Residential Care, 17*(5), 277-279. Retrieved on 19thDec 2016

fromhttp://www.magonlinelibrary.com/doi/abs/10.12968/nrec.2015.17.5.277

Ceccato, E., Vigato, G., Bonetto, C., Bevilacqua, A., Pizziolo, P., Crociani, S., & ... Barchi, E. (2012). STAM Protocol in Dementia: A Multicentre, Single-Blind, Randomized, and Controlled Trial. *American Journal of Alzheimer's Disease & Other Dementias, 27*(5), 301-310. doi:10.1177/1533317512452038

Chu, H., Yang, C., Lin, Y., Ou, K., Lee, T., O'Brien, A. P., & Chou, K. (2014). The Impact of Group Music Therapy on Depression and Cognition in Elderly Persons with Dementia: A Randomized Controlled Study. *Biological Research for Nursing, 16*(2), 209-217. doi:10.1177/1099800413485410

Cooke, M. L., Moyle, W., Shum, D. H., Harrison, S. D., & Murfield, J. E. (2010). A randomised controlled trial is exploring the effect of music on agitated behaviours and anxiety in older people with dementia. *Aging & Mental Health, 14*(8), 905-916. doi:10.1080/13607861003713190

Crotty,M. (1998). The foundations of social research, Sage Publications

Dementia Disease International, 2012. Retrieved on 13rdJan 2017 on

https://www.alz.co.uk/research/world-report-2012

Dementia: Music and the Mind Report, 2016.Retrieved on 19th Jan,

2017fromhttp://www.eldercarenet.org/blog/alzheimer2019s-dementia-music-and-the-mind

Denscombe, M. (2007). *The good research guide, for small-scale social research projects.* 3rdedition, Maidenhead: Open University Press.

Department of Health, 2005. *Research Governance Framework for Health and Social Care,* London: Department of Health.

Ellis, P. (2013). Understanding research for nursing students, 2nd Ed, London: Sage.

49

Goris, E. D., Ansel, K. N., & Schutte, D. L. (2016). Quantitative systematic review of the effects of non-pharmacological interventions on reducing apathy in persons with dementia. *Journal of Advanced Nursing, 72*(11), 2612-2628. doi:10.1111/jan.13026

Gray, D.E. (2014). *Doing research in the real world*, 3rd Ed, London: Sage.

Health and Social Care Information Centre (HSCIC), 2016. Retrieved on 15th Jan 2017 from http://content.digital.nhs.uk/catalogue/PUB19812/Focus-on-dementia-Jan-2016-v1-r1.pdf

Johnson, L., Deatrick, E. J., & Oriel, K. (2012). The Use of Music to Improve Exercise Participation in People with Dementia: A Pilot Study. *Physical & Occupational Therapy in Geriatrics, 30*(2), 102-108. doi:10.3109/02703181.2012.680008

Konno, R., Kang, H. S., & Makimoto, K. (2014). A best-evidence review of intervention studies for minimising resistance-to-care behaviours for older adults with dementia in nursing homes. *Journal of Advanced Nursing, 70*(10), 2167-2180. doi:10.1111/jan.12432

Leach, M. J., Francis, A., & Zairian, T. (2014). Improving the Health and Well-Being of Community-Dwelling Caregivers of Dementia Sufferers: Study Protocol of a Randomized Controlled Trial of Structured Meditation Training. *The Journal of Alternative and, Complementary Medicine 20*(2), 136-141. Retrieved on 19th Dec 2016 fromhttp://online.liebertpub.com/doi/pdf/10.1089/acm.2013.0170

Lin, Y., Chu, H., Yang, C., Chen, C., Chen, S., Chang, H., & ... Chou, K. (2011). Effectiveness of group music intervention against agitated behaviour in elderly persons with dementia. *International Journal of Geriatric Psychiatry, 26*(7), 670-678. doi:10.1002/gps.2580

Moher D, Liberati A, Tetzlaff J, Altman DG, The PRISMA Group (2009). *Preferred Reporting Items for Systematic Reviews and Meta-Analyses: The PRISMA Statement.* PLoS Med 6(7): e1000097. doi:10.1371/journal. pmed1000097

Murfield, J., Cooke, M., Moyle, W., Shum, D., & Harrison, S. (2011). Conducting randomised controlled trials with older people with dementia in long-term care: challenges and lessons learnt. *International Journal of Nursing Practice, 17*(1), 52-59. doi:10.1111/j.1440-172X.2010.

01906.x

Music Therapy Report, 2016.Retrieved on 19[th]Dec 2016

fromhttps://www.alz.org/cacentral/documents/Dementia_Care_9-

Music_Therapy_enhancing_cognition.pdf

Nair, B., Heim, C., Krishnan, C., D'Este, C., Marley, J., & Attia, J. (2011). The effect of Baroque

music on behavioural disturbances in patients with dementia. *Australasian Journal On*

Ageing, 30(1), 11-15. doi:10.1111/j.1741-6612.2010. 00439.x

Name, P., Clément, S., Ehrlé, N., Schiaratura, L., Vachez, S., Courtaigne, B., & ... Samson, S.

(2014). Efficacy of musical interventions in dementia: evidence from a randomised controlled

trial. *Journal of Alzheimer's Disease, 38*(1), 359-369. doi:10.3233/JAD-130893

NICE Guideline for quality assurance.Retrieved on 28th Aug 2017 from

http://www.scie.org.uk/publications/misc/dementia/dementia-fullguideline.pdf?res=true

O'Connor, C. M., Clemson, L., Brodaty, H., Gitlin, L. N., Piguet, O., & Mioshi, E. (2016).

Enhancing caregivers' understanding of dementia and tailoring activities in frontotemporal

dementia: two case studies. *Disability & Rehabilitation, 38*(7), 704-714.

doi:10.3109/09638288.2015.1055375

Parahoo, K. (2006). *Nursing research principles, process and issues*, Basingstoke: Palgrave

MacMillan.

PERSSON, G., & SKOOG, I. (1996). A prospective population study of psychosocial risk factors

for late onset dementia. *International Journal of Geriatric Psychiatry, 11*(1), 15-22. Retrieved on

19th Dec, 2016 from HTTP://onlinelibrary.wiley.com/doi/10.1002/(SICI)1099-

1166(199601)11:1%3C15::AID-GPS262%3E3.0.CO;2-5/full

Polit, D. F., & Beck, C. T. (2008). *Nursing research: Generating and assessing evidence for*

nursing practice. Lippincott Williams & Wilkins Retrieved on 15[th]Jan 2017 from

https://books.google.co.uk/books?hl=en&lr=&id=Ej3wstotgkQC&oi=fnd&pg=PA1&dq=Nursing+r

esearch+:+generating+and+assessing+evidence+for+nursing+practice+/+Denise+F.+Polit,+Ch

eryl+Tatano+Beck.&ots=wfQzFL5xDo&sig=TJcn8495nt3nDKs0k_JjuXtCZjw#v=onepage&q=Nu

rsing%20research%20%3A%20generating%20and%20assessing%20evidence%20for%20nursi

ng%20practice%20%2F%20Denise%20F.%20Polit%2C%20Cheryl%20Tatano%20Beck.&f=fals

e

Punch, K.F. (2014). Introduction to social research quantitative and qualitative approaches,

Sage: London.

Raglio, A., Bellandi, D., Baiardi, P., Gianotti, M., Ubezio, M. C., Zanacchi, E., & ... Stramba-

Badiale, M. (2015). Effect of Active Music Therapy and Individualized Listening to Music on

Dementia: A Multicentre Randomized Controlled Trial. *Journal of The American Geriatrics

Society, 63*(8), 1534-1539. doi:10.1111/jgs.13558

RCN. (2011). *Informed consent in health and social care research, RCN guidance for nurses,*

2nd Ed. Retrieved on 19th Dec, 2016 from RCN Website

http://www.rcn.org.uk/__data/assets/pdf_file/0010/78607/002267.pdf

Ridder, H. O., Stige, B., Qvale, L. G., & Gold, C. (2013). Individual music therapy for agitation in

dementia: an exploratory randomized controlled trial. *Aqinq & Mental Health, 17*(6), 667-678,

doi:10.1080/13607863.2013.790926

Ridley, D. (2012). *The literature review: A step-by-step guide for students.* Sage.Retrieved on

15th Jan, 2017 fromhttps://books.google.co.uk/books?hl=en&lr=&id=DF-

oJ0mstfEC&oi=fnd&pg=PP1&dq=ridley+doing+a++systematic+review+&ots=xQIP1IRJ3p&sig=

C0BpTHsr8dCxRvd8hdU4EUtByfw#v=onepage&q=ridley%20doing%20a%20%20systematic%2

0review&f=false

Rose, G. (2012). Visual Methodologies, an introduction to researching with visual materials, 3rd

Ed, London; Sage.

Särkämö, T., Laitinen, S., Numminen, A., Kurki, M., Johnson, J. K., & Rantanen, P. (2016).

Pattern of Emotional Benefits Induced by Regular Singing and Music Listening in

Dementia. *Journal of The American Geriatrics Society, 64*(2), 439-440. doi:10.1111/jgs.13963

Satizabal, C. L., Beiser, A. S., Chouraki, V., Chêne, G., Dufouil, C., & Seshadri, S. (2016).

Incidence of dementia over three decades in the Framingham Heart Study. *New England*

Journal of Medicine, 374(6), 523-532. Retrieved on 15th Jan, 2017 from

http://www.nejm.org/doi/full/10.1056/nejmoa1504327#t=article

Standring, S. (Ed.). (2015). *Gray's anatomy: the anatomical basis of clinical practice.* Elsevier

Health Sciences. Retrieved on 19th Dec, 2016

fromhttps://books.google.co.uk/books?hl=en&lr=&id=b7FVCgAAQBAJ&oi=fnd&pg=PP1&dq=Gr

ay%E2%80%99s+Anatomy,+2016&ots=4NmYJ1jGuw&sig=1emXGW24ByZRqjQJYfmlkoRphq

U#v=onepage&q=Gray%E2%80%99s%20Anatomy%2C%202016&f=false

Sung, H., Lee, W., Li, T., & Watson, R. (2012). A group music intervention using percussion

instruments with familiar music to reduce anxiety and agitation of institutionalized older adults

with dementia. *International Journal of Geriatric Psychiatry, 27*(6), 621-627.

doi:10.1002/gps.2761

University of Chester. (2014). *Research Governance Handbook,* retrieved on 15th Jan, 2017

from https://ganymede2.chester.ac.uk/view.php?title_id=522471

Van de Winckel, A., Fey, H., De Weerdt, W., & Dom, R. (2004). Cognitive and behavioural

effects of music-based exercises in patients with dementia. *Clinical Rehabilitation, 18*(3), 253-

260. Retrieved on 19th Dec, 2016 from https://www.ncbi.nlm.nih.gov/pubmed/15137556

Vink, A. C., Zuidersma, M., Boersma, F., Jonge, P., Zuidema, S. U., & Slaets, J. P. (2014).

Effect of Music Therapy Versus Recreational Activities on Neuropsychiatric Symptoms in Elderly

Adults with Dementia: An Exploratory Randomized Controlled Trial. *Journal of The American*

Geriatrics Society, 62(2), 392-393. doi:10.1111/jgs.12682

Watson R & Keady (2008) The nature and language of nursing. In: R Watson, H Mckenna, S

Cowman, J Keady, eds. Nursing Research. Churchill Livingstone Elsevier, Edinburgh. P3.

Watson, R., & Green, S. (2006). Feeding and dementia: a systematic literature review. *Journal*

of Advanced Nursing, 54(1), 86-93. doi:10.1111/j.1365-2648.2006. 03793.x

Wittwer, J. E., Webster, K. E., & Hill, K. (2013). Rhythmic auditory cueing to improve walking in

patients with neurological conditions other than Parkinson's disease - what is the

evidence. *Disability & Rehabilitation, 35*(2), 164-176. doi:10.3109/09638288.2012.690495

World Health Organization Factsheet, 2016. Retrieved on 19th Dec, 2016 from

http://www.who.int/mediacentre/factsheets/fs362/en/

World Health Organization Report, 2016. Retrieved on 25th Jan, 2017 from

http://www.who.int/gho/publications/world_health_statistics/en/

World Health Organization. (2012). *Dementia: a public health priority*. World Health

Organization. World Health Organization. (2012). *Dementia: a public health priority*. World

Health Organization. Retrieved on 25th Jan, 2017 from

https://www.cabdirect.org/cabdirect/abstract/20133159231

World Medical Association, (2013). Declaration of Helsinki. Retrieved on 15th Jan, 2017 from

http://www.wma.net/en/30publications/10policies/b3/

Yi-Hui, L., Shu-Ming, C., Man-Chun, C., & Tsuey-Yuan, H. (2014). The Use of Music

Intervention in Nursing Practice for Elderly Dementia Patients: A Systematic Review. *Journal of*

Nursing, 61(2), 84-94. doi:10.6224/JN.61.2.84

External References:

Buggey, T. (2007, Summer). A Picture Is Worth .... *Journal of Positive Behavior Interventions,*

9(3), 151-158. Retrieved December 14, 2007, from Academic Search Premier database.

Retrieved from

http://zh8wk8vq8w.search.serialssolutions.com/?genre=article&issn=13674676&title=The%20sp

irituality%20of%20people%20with%20late-

stage%20dementia:%20a%20review%20of%20the%20research%20literature,%20a%20critical

%20analysis%20and%20some%20implications%20for%20person-

centred%20spirituality%20and%20dementia%20care.&volume=18&issue=9&date=20151101&a

title=The%20spirituality%20of%20people%20with%20late-

stage%20dementia%3A%20a%20review%20of%20the%20research%20literature%2C%20a%2

0critical%20analysis%20and%20some%20implications%20for%20person-

centred%20spirituality%20and%20dementia%20care.&spage=765&pages=765-

776&sid=EBSCO:CINAHL%20Plus%20with%20Full%20Text&au=Kevern,%20Peter

Goris, E. D., Ansel, K. N., & Schutte, D. L. (2016). Quantitative systematic review of the effects

of non-pharmacological interventions on reducing apathy in persons with dementia. *Journal of

Advanced Nursing, 72*(11), 2612-2628. doi:10.1111/jan.13026

Johnson, L., Deatrick, E. J., & Oriel, K. (2012). The Use of Music to Improve Exercise

Participation in People with Dementia: A Pilot Study. *Physical & Occupational Therapy in

Geriatrics, 30*(2), 102-108. doi:10.3109/02703181.2012.680008

Konno, R., Kang, H. S., & Makimoto, K. (2014). A best-evidence review of intervention studies

for minimizing resistance-to-care behaviours for older adults with dementia in nursing

homes. *Journal of Advanced Nursing, 70*(10), 2167-2180. doi:10.1111/jan.12432

Lin, Y., Chu, H., Yang, C., Chen, C., Chen, S., Chang, H., & ... Chou, K. (2011). Effectiveness of

group music intervention against agitated behavior in elderly persons with

dementia. *International Journal of Geriatric Psychiatry, 26*(7), 670-678. doi:10.1002/gps.2580

Murfield, J., Cooke, M., Moyle, W., Shum, D., & Harrison, S. (2011). Conducting randomized

controlled trials with older people with dementia in long-term care: challenges and lessons

learnt. *International Journal of Nursing Practice, 17*(1), 52-59. doi:10.1111/j.1440-172X.2010.

01906.x

Raglio, A., Bellandi, D., Baiardi, P., Gianotti, M., Ubezio, M. C., Zanacchi, E., & ... Stramba-Badiale, M. (2015). Effect of Active Music Therapy and Individualized Listening to Music on Dementia: A Multicenter Randomized Controlled Trial. *Journal of The American Geriatrics Society, 63*(8), 1534-1539. doi:10.1111/jgs.13558

Sánchez, A., Maseda, A., Marante-Moar, M. P., de Labra, C., Lorenzo-López, L., & Millán-Calenti, J. C. (2016). Comparing the Effects of Multisensory Stimulation and Individualized Music Sessions on Elderly People with Severe Dementia: A Randomized Controlled Trial. *Journal of Alzheimer's Disease, 52*(1), 303-315. doi:10.3233/JAD-151150

Additional References:

Brett, L., Traynor, V., & Stapley, P. (2016). Effects of Physical Exercise on Health and Well-Being of Individuals Living with a Dementia in Nursing Homes: A Systematic Review. *Journal of The American Medical Directors Association, 17*(2), 104-116. doi: 10.1016/j.jamda.2015.08.016

Ceccato, E., Vigato, G., Bonetto, C., Bevilacqua, A., Pizziolo, P., Crociani, S., & ... Barchi, E. (2012). STAM Protocol in Dementia: A Multicenter, Single-Blind, Randomized, and Controlled Trial. *American Journal of Alzheimer's Disease & Other Dementias, 27*(5), 301-310. doi:10.1177/1533317512452038

Chu, H., Yang, C., Lin, Y., Ou, K., Lee, T., O'Brien, A. P., & Chou, K. (2014). The Impact of Group Music Therapy on Depression and Cognition in Elderly Persons with Dementia: A Randomized Controlled Study. *Biological Research for Nursing, 16*(2), 209-217. doi:10.1177/1099800413485410

Cooke, M. L., Moyle, W., Shum, D. H., Harrison, S. D., & Murfield, J. E. (2010). A randomized controlled trial exploring the effect of music on agitated behaviours and anxiety in older people with dementia. *Aging & Mental Health, 14*(8), 905-916. doi:10.1080/13607861003713190

Cooke, M., Moyle, W., Shum, D., Harrison, S., & Murfield, J. (2010). A randomized controlled trial exploring the effect of music on quality of life and depression in older people with dementia. *Journal of Health Psychology, 15*(5), 765-776. doi:10.1177/1359105310368188

Higgins, J. P., & Green, S. (Eds.). (2011). *Cochrane handbook for systematic reviews of interventions* (Vol. 4). John Wiley & Sons. Retrieved on 25th Jan, 2017 fromhttps://books.google.co.uk/books?hl=en&lr=&id=NKMg9sMM6GUC&oi=fnd&pg=PT13&dq= Higgins+and+Green,+2011&ots=LHZFOVDBI6&sig=OE7nWnOy2vhkhvz_YoeCohZPyvk#v=on epage&q=Higgins%20and%20Green%2C%202011&f=false

Brett, L., Traynor, V., & Stapley, P. (2016). Effects of Physical Exercise on Health and Well-Being of Individuals Living With a Dementia in Nursing Homes: A Systematic Review. *Journal of the American Medical Directors Association, 17*(2), 104-116. doi:10.1016/j.jamda.2015.08.016

Ceccato, E., Vigato, G., Bonetto, C., Bevilacqua, A., Pizziolo, P., Crociani, S., . . . Barchi, E. (2012). STAM Protocol in Dementia: A Multicenter, Single-Blind, Randomized, and Controlled Trial. *American Journal of Alzheimer's Disease & Other Dementias, 27*(5), 301-310. doi:10.1177/1533317512452038

Cheung, S. K. (2012). *The effects of the music-with-movement intervention of the cognitive functions of people with moderate dementia.* (Ph.D.), Hong Kong Polytechnic University (Hong Kong). Retrieved from http://search.ebscohost.com/login.aspx?direct=true&db=rzh&AN=109864009&site=ehost-live Available from EBSCOhost rzh database.

Chu, H., Yang, C.-Y., Lin, Y., Ou, K.-L., Lee, T.-Y., O'Brien, A. P., & Chou, K.-R. (2014). The Impact of Group Music Therapy on Depression and Cognition in Elderly Persons With Dementia: A Randomized Controlled Study. *Biological Research for Nursing, 16*(2), 209-217. doi:10.1177/1099800413485410

Cooke, M., Moyle, W., Shum, D., Harrison, S., & Murfield, J. (2010). A randomized controlled trial exploring the effect of music on quality of life and depression in older people with dementia. *Journal of Health Psychology, 15*(5), 765-776. doi:10.1177/1359105310368188

Cooke, M. L., Moyle, W., Shum, D. H. K., Harrison, S. D., & Murfield, J. E. (2010). A randomized controlled trial exploring the effect of music on agitated behaviours and anxiety in older people with dementia. *Aging & Mental Health, 14*(8), 905-916. doi:10.1080/13607861003713190

Eun-Hi, K., & Myonghwa, P. (2015). Effects of Music Therapy on Agitation in Dementia: Systematic Review and Meta-analysis. *Korean Journal of Adult Nursing, 27*(1), 106-116. doi:10.7475/kjan.2015.27.1.106

Goris, E. D., Ansel, K. N., & Schutte, D. L. (2016). Quantitative systematic review of the effects of non-pharmacological interventions on reducing apathy in persons with dementia. *Journal of Advanced Nursing, 72*(11), 2612-2628. doi:10.1111/jan.13026

Han, J. W., Lee, H., Hong, J. W., Kim, K., Kim, T., Byun, H. J., . . . Kim, K. W. (2017). Multimodal Cognitive Enhancement Therapy for Patients with Mild Cognitive Impairment and Mild Dementia: A Multi- Center, Randomized, Controlled, Double-Blind, Crossover Trial. *Journal of Alzheimer's Disease. 55*(2). 787-796.

Harrison, S., Cooke, M., Moyle, W., Shum, D., & Murfield, J. E. (2010). Development of a music intervention protocol and its effect on participant engagement: experiences from a randomised controlled trial with older people with dementia. *Arts & Health: International Journal for Research, Policy & Practice, 2*(2), 125-139. doi:10.1080/17533015.2010.490839

Holmes, C., Knights, A., Dean, C., Hodkinson, S., Hopkins, V., Holmes, C., . . . Hopkins, V. (2006). Keep music live: music and the alleviation of apathy in dementia subjects. *International Psychogeriatrics, 18*(4), 623-630.

Johnson, L., Deatrick, E. J., & Oriel, K. (2012). The Use of Music to Improve Exercise

Participation in People with Dementia: A Pilot Study. *Physical & Occupational Therapy in*

Geriatrics, 30(2), 102-108. doi:10.3109/02703181.2012.680008

Konno, R., Kang, H. S., & Makimoto, K. (2014). A best-evidence review of intervention studies

for minimizing resistance-to-care behaviours for older adults with dementia in nursing homes.

Journal of Advanced Nursing, 70(10), 2167-2180. doi:10.1111/jan.12432

Lin, Y., Chu, H., Yang, C.-Y., Chen, C.-H., Chen, S.-G., Chang, H.-J., . . . Chou, K.-R. (2011).

Effectiveness of group music intervention against agitated behavior in elderly persons with

dementia. *International Journal of Geriatric Psychiatry, 26*(7), 670-678. doi:10.1002/gps.2580

Livingston, G., & Lim, L. S. (2015). 2014 - Review: In patients with dementia who live in care

homes, some nondrug interventions reduce agitation. *ACP Journal Club, 162*(12), 1-1.

doi:10.7326/ACPJC-2015-162-12-003

Matthews, S. (2015). Dementia and the Power of Music Therapy. *Bioethics, 29*(8), 573-579.

doi:10.1111/bioe.12148

McDermott, O., Orrell, M., & Ridder, H. M. (2015). The development of Music in Dementia

Assessment Scales (MiDAS). *Nordic Journal of Music Therapy, 24*(3), 232-251.

doi:10.1080/08098131.2014.907333

McHugh, L., Gardstrom, S., Hiller, J., Brewer, M., & Diestelkamp, W. S. (2012). The Effect of

Pre-Meal, Vocal Re-Creative Music Therapy on Nutritional Intake of Residents with Alzheimer's

Disease and Related Dementias: A Pilot Study. *Music Therapy Perspectives, 30*(1), 32-42.

Mendes, A. (2015). 'Unlocking' people with dementia through the use of music therapy. *Nursing*

& Residential Care, 17(9), 512-514.

Nair, B., Heim, C., Krishnan, C., D'Este, C., Marley, J., & Attia, J. (2011). The effect of Baroque

music on behavioural disturbances in patients with dementia. *Australasian Journal on Ageing,*

30(1), 11-15. doi:10.1111/j.1741-6612.2010.00439.x

Narme, P., Clément, S., Ehrlé, N., Schiaratura, L., Vachez, S., Courtaigne, B., . . . Samson, S. (2014). Efficacy of musical interventions in dementia: evidence from a randomized controlled trial. *Journal of Alzheimer's Disease, 38*(1), 359-369. doi:10.3233/JAD-130893

Pavlicevic, M., Tsiris, G., Wood, S., Powell, H., Graham, J., Sanderson, R., . . . Gibson, J. (2015). The 'ripple effect': Towards researching improvisational music therapy in dementia care homes. *Dementia (14713012), 14*(5), 659-679. doi:10.1177/1471301213514419

Quach, J. (2017). Do music therapies reduce depressive symptoms and improve QOL in older adults with chronic disease? *Nursing, 47*(6), 58-63. doi:10.1097/01.NURSE.0000513604.41152.0c

Raglio, A., Bellandi, D., Baiardi, P., Gianotti, M., Ubezio, M. C., Zanacchi, E., . . . Stramba-Badiale, M. (2015). Effect of Active Music Therapy and Individualized Listening to Music on Dementia: A Multicenter Randomized Controlled Trial. *Journal of the American Geriatrics Society, 63*(8), 1534-1539. doi:10.1111/jgs.13558

Ray, K. D., & Mittelman, M. S. (2017). Music therapy: A nonpharmacological approach to the care of agitation and depressive symptoms for nursing home residents with dementia. *Dementia (14713012), 16*(6), 689-710. doi:10.1177/1471301215613779

Ridder, H. M. O., Stige, B., Qvale, L. G., & Gold, C. (2013). Individual music therapy for agitation in dementia: an exploratory randomized controlled trial. *Aging & Mental Health, 17*(6), 667-678. doi:10.1080/13607863.2013.790926

Sánchez, A., Maseda, A., Marante-Moar, M. P., de Labra, C., Lorenzo-López, L., & Millán-Calenti, J. C. (2016). Comparing the Effects of Multisensory Stimulation and Individualized Music Sessions on Elderly People with Severe Dementia: A Randomized Controlled Trial. *Journal of Alzheimer's Disease, 52*(1), 303-315. doi:10.3233/JAD-151150

Särkämö, T., Laitinen, S., Numminen, A., Kurki, M., Johnson, J. K., & Rantanen, P. (2016). Clinical and Demographic Factors Associated with the Cognitive and Emotional Efficacy of

Regular Musical Activities in Dementia. *Journal of Alzheimer's Disease, 49*(3), 767-781.

doi:10.3233/JAD-150453

Särkämö, T., Laitinen, S., Numminen, A., Kurki, M., Johnson, J. K., & Rantanen, P. (2016).

Pattern of Emotional Benefits Induced by Regular Singing and Music Listening in Dementia

(Vol. 64, pp. 439-440). Malden, Massachusetts: Wiley-Blackwell.

Seitz, D. P., Brisbin, S., Herrmann, N., Rapoport, M. J., Wilson, K., Gill, S. S., . . . Conn, D.

(2012). Efficacy and Feasibility of Nonpharmacological Interventions for Neuropsychiatric

Symptoms of Dementia in Long Term Care: A Systematic Review. *Journal of the American

Medical Directors Association, 13*(6), 503-506.e502. doi:10.1016/j.jamda.2011.12.059

Sung, H., Chang, S., Lee, W., & Lee, M. (2006). The effects of group music with movement

intervention on agitated behaviours of institutionalized elders with dementia in Taiwan.

Complementary Therapies in Medicine, 14(2), 113-119.

Sung, H. C., Lee, W. L., Li, T. L., & Watson, R. (2012). A group music intervention using

percussion instruments with familiar music to reduce anxiety and agitation of institutionalized

older adults with dementia. *International Journal of Geriatric Psychiatry, 27*(6), 621-627.

doi:10.1002/gps.2761

Spiro, N., Farrant, C. L., & Pavlicevic, M. (2017). Between practice, policy and politics: Music

therapy and the Dementia Strategy, 2009. *Dementia (14713012), 16*(3), 259-281.

doi:10.1177/1471301215585465

Van de Winckel, A., Fey, H., De Weerdt, W., & Dom, R. (2004). Cognitive and behavioural

effects of music-based exercises in patients with dementia. *Clinical Rehabilitation, 18*(3), 253-

260.

Vasionytė, I., & Madison, G. (2013). Musical intervention for patients with dementia: a meta-

analysis. *Journal of Clinical Nursing, 22*(9/10), 1203-1216. doi:10.1111/jocn.12166

Vink, A. C., Zuidersma, M., Boersma, F., Jonge, P., Zuidema, S. U., & Slaets, J. P. (2014). Effect of Music Therapy Versus Recreational Activities on Neuropsychiatric Symptoms in Elderly Adults with DementiA: An Exploratory Randomized Controlled Trial. *Journal of the American Geriatrics Society, 62*(2), 392-393. doi:10.1111/jgs.12682

Watson, R., & Green, S. M. (2006). Feeding and dementia: a systematic literature review. *Journal of Advanced Nursing, 54*(1), 86-93. doi:10.1111/j.1365-2648.2006.03793.x

Werner, J., Wosch, T., & Gold, C. (2017). Effectiveness of group music therapy versus recreational group singing for depressive symptoms of elderly nursing home residents: pragmatic trial. *Aging & Mental Health, 21*(2), 147-155. doi:10.1080/13607863.2015.1093599

Yi-Hui, L., Shu-Ming, C., Man-Chun, C., & Tsuey-Yuan, H. (2014). The Use of Music Intervention in Nursing Practice for Elderly Dementia Patients: A Systematic Review. *Journal of Nursing, 61*(2), 84-94. doi:10.6224/JN.61.2.84

Yu-Shiun, C., Hsin, C., Chyn-Yng, Y., Jui-Chen, T., Min-Huey, C., Yuan-Mei, L., . . . Kuei-Ru, C. (2015). The efficacy of music therapy for people with dementia: A meta-analysis of randomised controlled trials. *Journal of Clinical Nursing, 24*(23/24), 3425-3440. doi:10.1111/jocn.12976

Key References

Blaxter, L., Hughes, C., & Tight, M. (2006). *How to research* (3rd ed.). Buckingham: Open University Press.

Bowling, A., & Ebrahim, S. (2005). Handbook of health research methods: Investigation, measurement and analysis. Berkshire: Open University Press.

Bryman, A. (2008). *Social research methods* (3rd ed.). Oxford: Oxford University Press.

Hart, C. (2001). Doing a literature search: a comprehensive guide for the social sciences. London: Sage Publications.

Hart, C. (2005). *Doing your Masters dissertation.* London: Sage Publications.

Oliver, P. (2003). *The student's guide to research ethics.* Maidenhead: Open University Press/McGraw Hill.

Oliver, P. (2008). *Writing your thesis* (2nd ed.). London: Sage Publications.

Phelps, R., Fisher, K., & Ellis, A. (2007). Organising and managing your research: A practical guide for postgraduates. London: Sage Publications.

Punch, K. F. (2006). *Developing effective research proposals* (2nd ed.). London: Sage Publications.

Rudestam, K., & Newton, R. (2007). Surviving your dissertation: A comprehensive guide to content and process. (3rd ed.). London: Sage Publications

Reference List for Ethical Approval:

Beauchamp, T., Childress, J. (2008). *Principles of biomedical ethics*, 6th Ed, Oxford University Press: Oxford.

Bowling,A. (2014). Research methods in health, investigating health and health services, 4th Ed, Open University Press: Maidenhead

British Economic and Social Research Council (ESRC). (2012). *Framework for research ethics*, retrieved from http://www.esrc.ac.uk/about-esrc/information/research-ethics.aspx

Department of Health.(2005). *Research Governance Framework for Health and Social Care*, London: Department of Health.

Denscombe,M.(2007). *The good research guide, for small-scale social research projects.* 3rdedition, Maidenhead: Open University Press.

Ellis,P. (2013). Understanding research for nursing students, 2nd Ed, London: Sage.

Gray, D.E. (2014). *Doing research in the real world*, 3rd Ed, London: Sage.

Office of Public Sector Information.(1998). *Data protection act*, ch 29.London:HMSO.

Parahoo, K.(2006). *Nursing research principles, process and issues*, Basingstoke: Palgrave MacMillan.

Pink, S.(2007).*Doing visual ethnography*, Sage publications: London.

Punch,K.F.(2014). Introduction to social research quantitative and qualitative approaches, Sage: London.

RCN. (2011). *Informed consent in health and social care research, RCN guidance for nurses*, 2nd Ed, retrieved from RCN Website

http://www.rcn.org.uk/__data/assets/pdf_file/0010/78607/002267.pdf

Rose, G. (2012). Visual Methodologies, an introduction to researching with visual materials, 3rd Ed, London; Sage.

University of Chester. (2014). *Research Governance Handbook*, retrieved from

https://ganymede2.chester.ac.uk/view.php?title_id=522471

Wiles,R., Clark, A., Prosser, J. (2011). *Visual Research Ethics at the crossroads* in Margolis, E., Pauwels, L. (eds). (2011). The sage handbook of visual research methods, (pp 685-706), Sage: London.

WMA. (2013). Declaration of Helsinki. Retrieved from

http://www.wma.net/en/30publications/10policies/b3/

APPENDIX: 1:

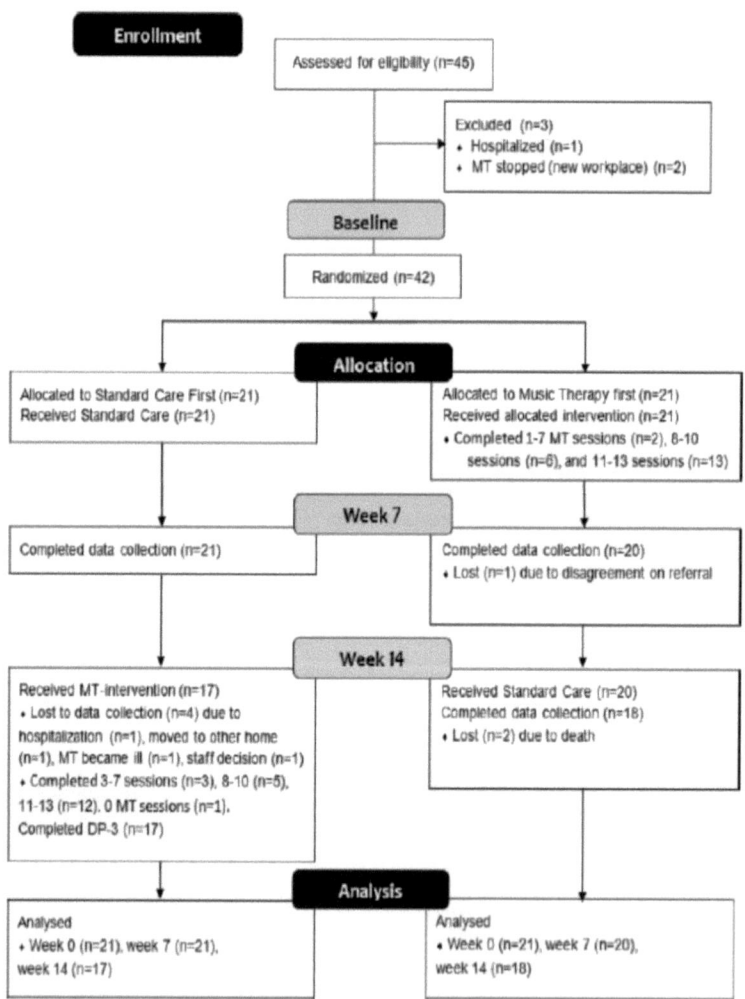

Participant flow (CONSORT).

Appendix: 2:

Plan: Systematic Review:

Title	A systematic review on the effect of music therapy on cognitive and behavioural function of older adults with dementia
Abstract	Content that will be included in the abstract: • Objective • sample and setting • Methods • Data collection and analysis • Results/Findings • Conclusion keywords
Background	Criteria for considering studies: Dementia is a rising global health issue stated by World Health Organisation's factsheet of April, 2016 as follows: • Dementia is a syndrome in which there is deterioration in memory, thinking, behaviour and the ability to perform everyday activities. • Although dementia mainly affects older people, it is not a normal part of ageing. • Worldwide, 47.5 million people have dementia and there are 7.7 million new cases every year. • Alzheimer's disease is the common type of dementia whichcomprises of 60–70% of total dementia patients (WHO Report, 2016) • Dementia is one of the major causes of disability and dependency among older people worldwide.

	• Dementia has physical, psychological, social and economic impact on caregivers, families and society. Condition/ Disease: Dementia Intervention: Music therapy How the intervention might work: By stimulating the neuron by cognitive therapy e.g. music therapy which will help the older adults to recover their previous memories Why it is important to do this review: to increase the strength of the previous randomised control trials by accumulating the results of all RCTs in a systematic review. It will be beneficial for the older age group if this study shows positive association between increase cognitive function of the patients by using music therapy on a regular basis
Objectives	Precise statement of the primary aim: -To evaluate the effect of music therapy on cognitive functions of older adult patients with dementia - To evaluate the effect of music therapy on behavioural functions of older adult patients with dementia
Methods	• Search strategy: by gathering all randomised control trials from all available search engines via website e.g. Cochrane, CINAHL, PUBMED, etc. by using PRIXMA statement (Moher D, Liberati A, Tetzlaff J, Altman DG, The PRISMA Group, 2009). Methods of the review (selection of studies, data extraction and management, quality assessment and data analysis):

Methods: Inclusion/ exclusion criteria

- Research Design: Randomised Control Trials (RCTs)

- Research Sample size: Gathering all the samples of all related RCTs

- Participants: Older adults with dementia and involved in music therapy

- Settings: Regardless of all RCTs settings

- Quality assurance/ethical issue: For quality control, critical review of ethical approval will be done and ethical approval (Boland et al., 2008) from the authority will be done before starting the systematic review

- Data collection procedure/technique: gathering all randomised control trials from all available search engines via data extraction tables anddatabases e.g. Cochrane, CINAHL, PUBMED, etc.

- Data analysis: thematic analysis for qualitative data, RevMan version 5.0 for quantitative data will be used to do the meta-analysis to analyse all the RCT results

Results	Outline how you will present the results (description of studies):
	-results will be presented as diagram, table, pie charts, bar charts, etc from MS Excel or RevMan, PRIXMA Flow Chart, etc.
	Presentation of included studies and excluded studies:
	Included studies:
	Those studies which shows randomised control trials on dementia patients who is older adults and taking music therapies
	Excluded studies:
	Dementia patient who is older adults taking other therapies than the music therapy
	Brief summary of the papers methodological quality: - Randomised control trials based papers will be selected only for doing the systematic review as we all know that Randomised control trials are the gold standard of all studies, but because of small sample size of these Randomised control trials, the result is not as much as strong as a systematic review

	- For quality control of ethical issues, critical review of ethical approval will be done and ethical approval from the authority will be done before starting the systematic review Provide an overview of the actual results: There might be some positive effects on older adults by involving with the music therapy which will help them to reconnect with their previous neurons effectively. That is how, music therapy might help them by increasing their cognitive level and behavioural habits by listening to their favourite previous music
Conclusion	- Outline for the full systematic review will be provided in the end of the proposal - Recommendations - References: Recommended APA referencing style will be followed - Appendices - Time schedule

Appendix: 4: (Figures)

Predicted Aging population with Dementia by 2051:

(Health and Social Care Information Centre, 2016)

Background – an ageing population

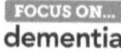

dementia

The risk of developing dementia increases as people age. The increase in the older population over recent decades is projected to continue. As the older population increases we would expect see a similar increase in the number of dementia cases unless the incidence of new dementia cases decreases.

Growth is forecast in all older age groups. By 2051, as many as one in four people (25 per cent) will be aged 65 or over and one in 15 people (7 per cent) aged 85 or over.

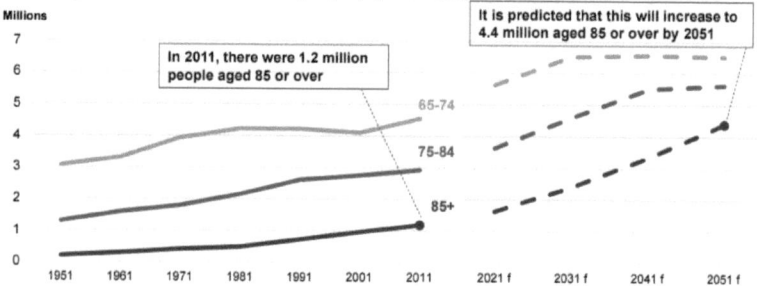

Figure 0: Predicted aged population with Dementia by 2051

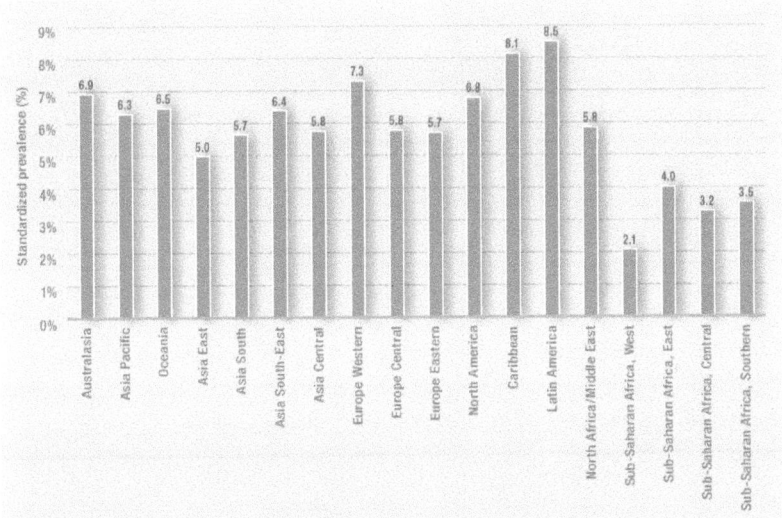

FIG 2.2 Estimated prevalence of dementia for persons aged 60 and over, standardized to Western Europe population, by Global Burden of Disease region

Figure 6: WHO Report, 2016: Global Burden of Disease due to Dementia

GBD region	Population over 60 years (millions, 2010)	Crude estimated prevalence (%, 2010)	Number of people with dementia (millions)			Proportionate increases (%)	
			2010	2030	2050	2010–2030	2010–2050
ASIA	406.55	3.9	15.94	33.04	60.92	107	282
Australasia	4.82	6.4	0.31	0.53	0.79	71	157
Asia Pacific	46.63	6.1	2.83	5.36	7.03	89	148
Oceania	0.49	4.0	0.02	0.04	0.10	100	400
Asia, Central	7.16	4.6	0.33	0.56	1.19	70	261
Asia, East	171.61	3.2	5.49	11.93	22.54	117	311
Asia, South	124.61	3.6	4.48	9.31	18.12	108	304
Asia, Southeast	51.22	4.8	2.48	5.30	11.13	114	349
EUROPE	160.18	6.2	9.95	13.95	18.65	40	87
Europe, Western	97.27	7.2	6.98	10.03	13.44	44	93
Europe, Central	23.61	4.7	1.10	1.57	2.10	43	91
Europe, East	39.30	4.8	1.87	2.36	3.10	26	66
THE AMERICAS	120.74	6.5	7.82	14.78	27.08	89	246
North America	63.67	6.9	4.38	7.13	11.01	63	151
Caribbean	5.06	6.5	0.33	0.62	1.04	88	215
Latin America, Andean	4.51	5.6	0.25	0.59	1.29	136	416
Latin America, Central	19.54	6.1	1.19	2.79	6.37	134	435
Latin America, Southern	8.74	7.0	0.61	1.08	1.83	77	200
Latin America, Tropical	19.23	5.5	1.05	2.58	5.54	146	428

Figure 7: Total population over 60yrs, prevalence of dementia(2010): Global burden of Dementia, WHO, 2016

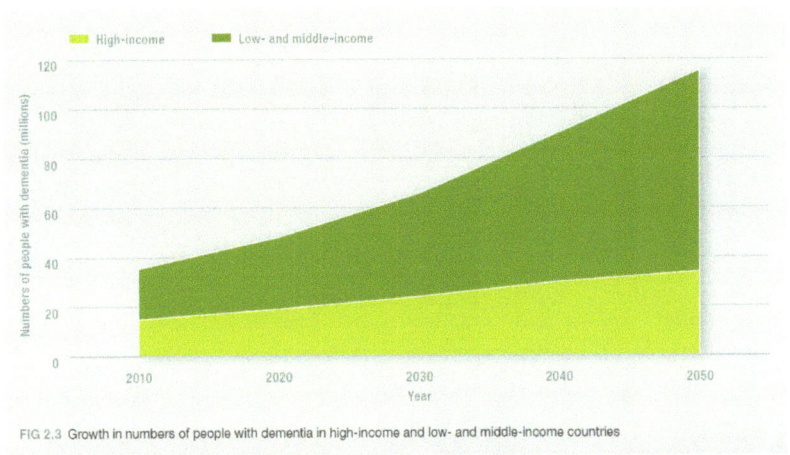

FIG 2.3 Growth in numbers of people with dementia in high-income and low- and middle-income countries

Figure 8: GROWTH IN NO. OF PEOPLE WITH DEMENTIA IN DIFFERENT COUNTRY SETTING (WHO, 2016)

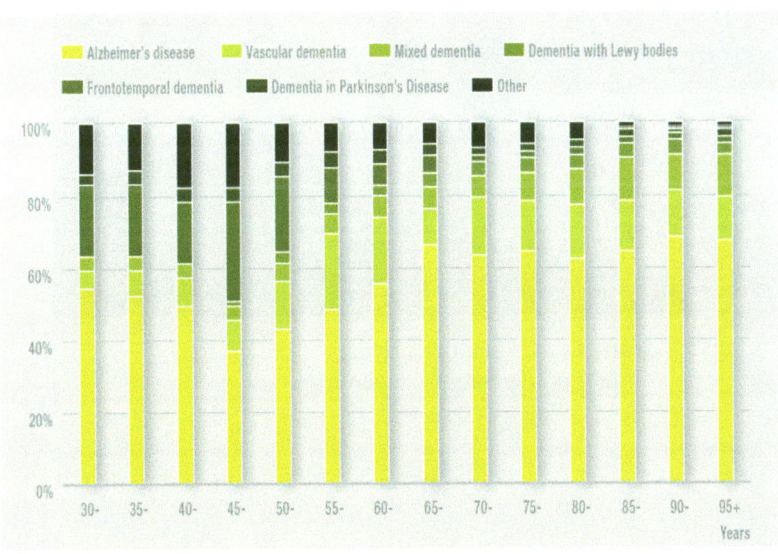

Figure 9: Different types of dementia in Women(WHO, 2016)

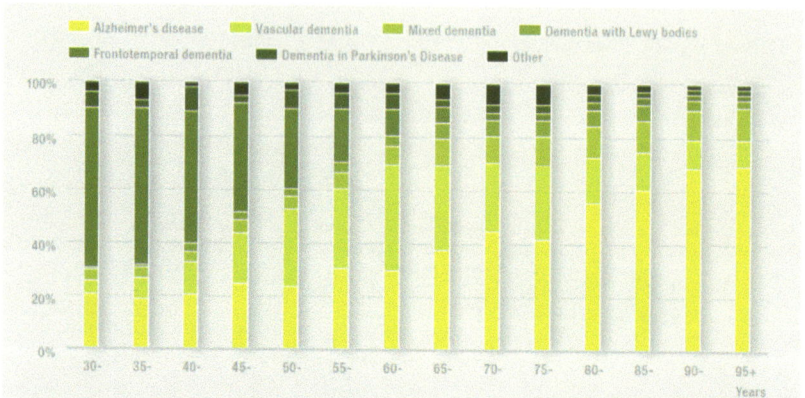

Figure 10: Different types of dementia in Men(WHO, 2016)

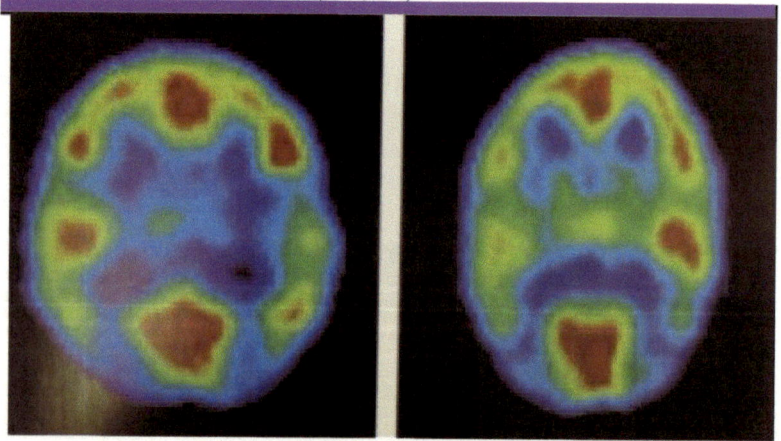

PET-scans showing brain activity in speech (left)
and in listening to music (right).

Figure 6: Braining activity during music therapy and Speech (PET CT Scan). Red areas: anger during speech

Appendix 5:

PICO

PICO framework is used to develop literature searching strategies:

P – patient, problem or population

I – intervention

C – comparison, control or comparator[5]

O – outcome

SCREENING/ SELECTION TOOL

STUDY ID	Registered ID for doing the systematic review	
PICO	Inclusion Variables	Response (will be evaluated during the dissertation process)
Review Question	To evaluate the effect of music therapy on cognitive functions of older adult patients with dementia and to evaluate the effect of music therapy on behavioral functions of older adult patients with dementia in the United Kingdom	
Population	Dementia patients who is older adults (45 to 69 years old) and taking music therapies in Randomized control trials (RCTs)	
Intervention	a. music therapies	
Comparator	a. Placebo group of other randomized control trials	

Outcome	a. Dementia improvement in cognitive and behavioral functions of older adult patients with dementia	
Setting	a. Hospital b. Bar c. Club d. Any other registered area for the therapy	
Study Design	Level A, B & C evidence based studies such as: a. Systematic reviews b. Randomized Controlled Trials c. Cohort studies	

(Boland et al, 2013)

Appendix 6:

PRISMA FLOW DIAGRAM

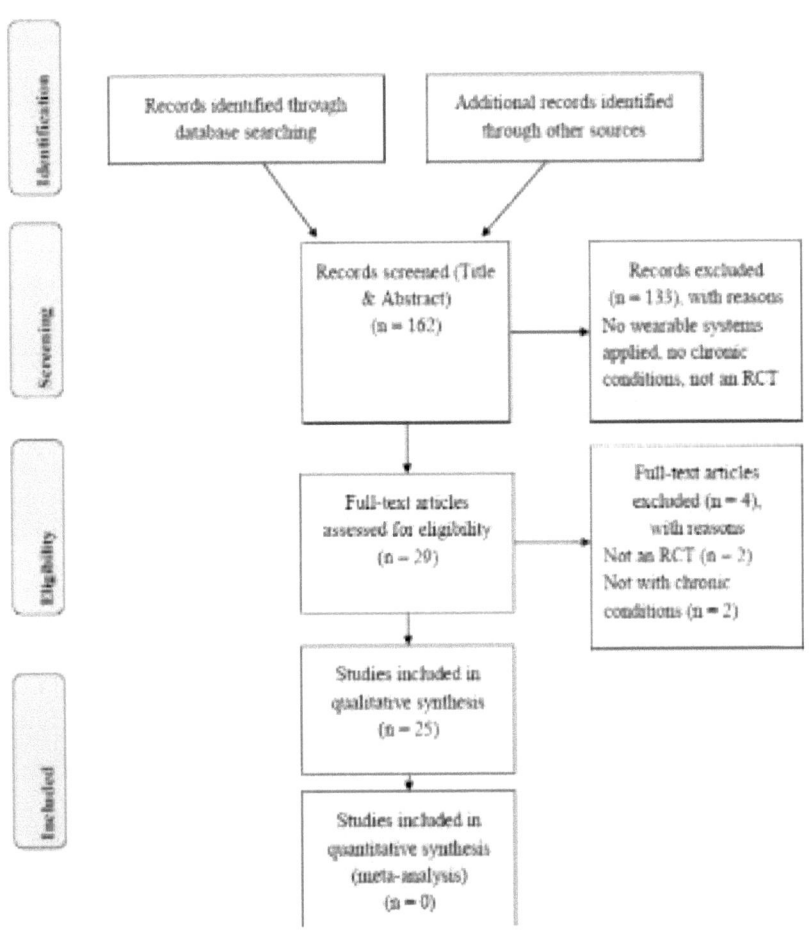

APPENDIX:7:

Quality and Critical Appraisal of Included Studies

Table: CASP Checklist

S/N	Author	1	2	3	4	5	6	7	8	9	10	11
1	Ceccato, et al. 2012	Y	Y	Y	Y	Y	Y	Significant difference between study groups in getting music therapy	Y	Y	Y	Y
2	The Chu, et al. 2013	Y	Y	Y	Y	Y	Y	There was a significant reduction of dementia in both groups	Y	Y	Y	Y
3	Cooke, et al. 2010	Y	Y	Y	Y	Y	Y	Moderate reduction in the music therapy indices in the intervention group	Y	Y	Y	Y

4	Konno, Kang, & Makimoto, 2014	Y	Y	Y	Y	Y	Y	No significant change in intervention group				
5	Leach, Francis, & Ziaian,2014	Y	Y	Y	Y	Y	Y	Dementia indices did not differ significantly between the two groups with or without the Intervention	Y	Y	Y	Y
6	Brett, Traynor, & Stapley, 2016	Y	Y	Y	Y	Y	Y	Result show moderate reduction in dementia	Y	Y	Y	Y
7	Lin, et al. 2011	Y	Y	Y	Y	Y	Y	Significant improvement in dementia patients in randomized control trial	Y	Y	Y	Y
8	Murfield, Cooke,	Y	Y	Y	Y	Y	Y	Significant reduction in	Y	Y	Y	Y

	Moyle, Shum, & Harrison, 2011							the clinical incidence of dementia after the therapy				
9	Nair, Heim, Krishnan, D'Este, Marley, & Attia, 2011	Y	Y	Y	Y	Y	Y	No statistically significant difference between the protective efficacies of the intervention group	Y	Y	Y	Y
10	Raglio et al., 2015	Y	Y	Y	Y	Y	Y	Significant improvement of dementia in music therapy groups	Y	Y	Y	Y
11	Ridder, Stige, Qvale, & Gold,2013	Y	Y	Y	Y	Y	Y	Significant improvement of dementia in music	Y	Y	Y	Y

								therapy group				
12	Sánchez, et al., 2016	Y	Y	Y	Y	Y	Y	Significant improvement of dementia in music therapy group	Y	Y	Y	Y
13	Vink, Zuidersma, Boersma, Jonge, Zuidema, & Slaets, 2014	Y	Y	Y	Y	Y	Y	Significant improvement of dementia in music therapy groups	Y	Y	Y	Y

Appendex:8: Timeline of this Systematic Review Research:

Graphical representation:

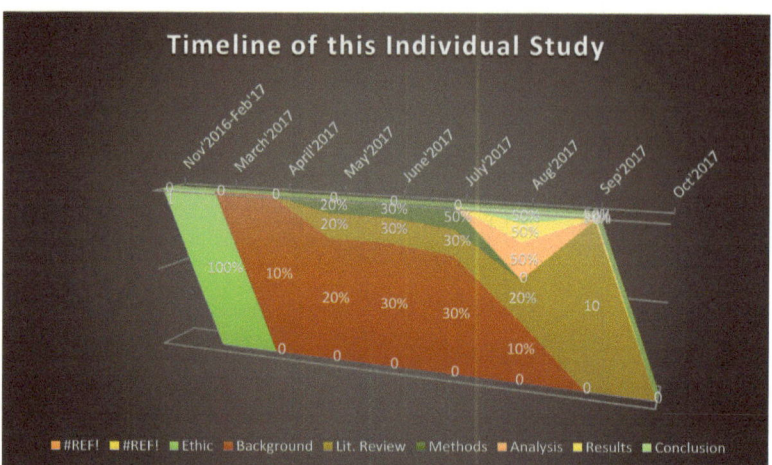

Table:

TIME PERIOD	WORK
Feb – April, 2017	Reviewing the literatures/RCTs again Reviewingthe research questions Carrying out further literature searches Pilot testing
May-June, 2017	Literature Searches and Data collection from the previous RCT
May-June, 2017	Screening for Inclusion
May-June, 2017	Validity assessment of the included studies

July-Aug, 2017	Thematic analysis and RevMan analysis
July-Aug, 2017	Chasing for missing information/ studies
Sep-Oct, 2017	Writing up the whole dissertation's finding and conclusion
7thNov 2017	Submission to Turnitin

Appendix:9:

Levels of evidence based studies

EVIDENCE BASED LEVELS	TYPE OF RESEARCH OR STUDY
Level A	Highest quality of: 'Systematic Review' 'Randomized Controlled Trials 'Cohort stu.dy.'
Level B	Limited: 'Systematic Review" 'Randomized Controlled Trials 'Cohort stu.dy.'
Level C	Case control study
Level D	Case series Limited Cohort Case control study
Level E	Expert opinion

(Bateman, Barclay and Saunders, 2010)

Appendex:10:

Checklist for Data Collection & Extraction:

(Higgins and Green, 2011):

SOURCE	• Study ID • Report ID • Review author ID • Citation and contact details
ELIGIB ILITY	• Confirm eligibility for review • Reason for exclusion
METHODS	• Study design • Total study duration • Allocation sequence concealment • Blinding • Other concerns about bias
PARTICIPANTS	• Total number • Setting • Diagnostic criteria • Age • Sex • Country • Date of study

INTERVENTIONS	• Total number of intervention groups For each intervention and comparison group of interest: • Specific intervention • Intervention details
OUTCOME	• Outcomes and time points (i) collected; (ii) reported For each outcome of interest: • Outcome definition (with diagnostic criteria) • Unit of measurement (if relevant) • For scales: upper and lower limits, and whether high or low score is good
RESULTS	• Number of participants allocated to each intervention group For each outcome of interest: • Sample size • Missing participants • Summary data for each intervention group (e.g. 2×2 table for dichotomous data; means and SDs for continuous data) • Estimate of effect with confidence interval; P value • Subgroup analyses

MISCELLANEOUS	• Funding source
	• Key conclusions of the study authors
	• Miscellaneous comments from the study authors
	• References to other relevant studies
	• Correspondence required

(Higgins and Green, 2011)

APPENDIX:11

SUMMARY OF THE RESULTS OF QUALITY ASSESSMENT FOR RANDOMISED CONTROLLED STUDIES

Study	Truly random	Allocation	Number stated	Presented	Achieved	Inclusion criteria	Co-intervention	Assessors	Administration	Participants	Procedure assessed	>80% n final analysis	Reasons stated	Intention to treat	Other outcome

NS: Not Suitable   NA: Not Applicable   ✓ :   Item adequately addressed ✗   :

Item not adequately addressed

(Boland et al, 2001)

SUMMARY OF THE RESULTS OF QUALITY ASSESSMENT FOR NON- RANDOMISED

CONTROLLED STUDIES FOR THE NEWCASTLE- OTTAWA ASSESSMENT TOOL

(TOTAL NO OF STARS ATTAINED BY EACH STUDY)

STUDY ID	SELECTION	COMPARITIBILITY	EXPOSURE

(Author' own work)

VALIDITY AND QUALITY OF ALL INCLUDED STUDIES

No.	Study	Allocation	Blinding	Follow up & exclusions	Selective reporting	Other sources of potential bias
1						
2						
3						
4						
5						
6						
7						
8						
9						
10						

(Boland et al, 2001)

Entry	Judgement High/ Low	Support for Judgement
Random sequence generation (selection bias)		Quote: Comment:
Allocation concealment (selection bias)		Quote: Comment:
Blinding of participants and personnel (performance bias)		Quote: Comment:
Blinding of outcome assessment (detection bias) (patient-reported outcomes)		Quote: Comment:
Blinding of outcome		

assessment (detection bias) (Mortality)		
Incomplete outcome data addressed (attrition bias) (Short-term outcomes (2-6 weeks))		
Incomplete outcome data addressed (attrition bias) (Longer-term outcomes (>6 weeks))		
Selective reporting (reporting bias)		

CATEGORIZING RISK CATEGORY FOR THE STUDIES

(Higgins and Green, 2011)

RECORD OF ALL SHORTLISTED STUDIES

No	Reference	Included at screening	Obtained paper	Included at selection
1				
2				
3				
4				
5				
6				
7				
8				
9				
10				

(Boland et al, 2001)

QA TOOL FOR SYSTEMATIC REVIEW

No.	Quality Item	Response
	Was the review question clearly defined in terms of population, intervention, comparators, outcome and study designs?	
	Was the search strategy adequate and appropriate?	
	Were preventative steps taken to minimize bias and errors in the study selection process?	

Were appropriate criteria used to assess the quality of the primary studies, and preventative steps taken to minimize bias and errors in the quality assessment process?	
Were preventative steps taken to minimize bias and errors in the data extraction process?	
Were appropriate methods used for data synthesis?	
Were differences between studies assessed?	
Were the studies pooled, and if so was it appropriate and meaningful to do so?	
Do the authors' conclusions accurately reflect the evidence that was reviewed?	

NS: Not Suitable   NA: Not Applicable ✓ :   Item adequately addressed ✗ : Item not adequately addressed

(Boland et al, 2001)

APPENDIX: TABLES

CLASSIFICATION FOR BIAS

Type of bias	Description	Relevant domains in the Collaboration's 'Risk of bias' tool
Selection bias	Systematic differences between baseline characteristics of the groups that are compared.	Sequence generation. Allocation concealment.
Performance bias	Systematic differences between groups in the care that is provided, or in exposure to factors other than the interventions of interest.	• Blinding of participants and personnel. • Other potential threats to validity.

Detection bias	Systematic differences between groups in how outcomes are determined.	• Blinding of outcome assessment. • Other potential threats to validity.
Attrition bias	Systematic differences between groups in withdrawals from a study.	• Incomplete outcome data
Reporting bias	Systematic differences between reported and unreported findings.	• Selective outcome reporting

(Higgins and Green, 2011)

Search strategy and study selection: (PRISMA FLOW DIAGRAM

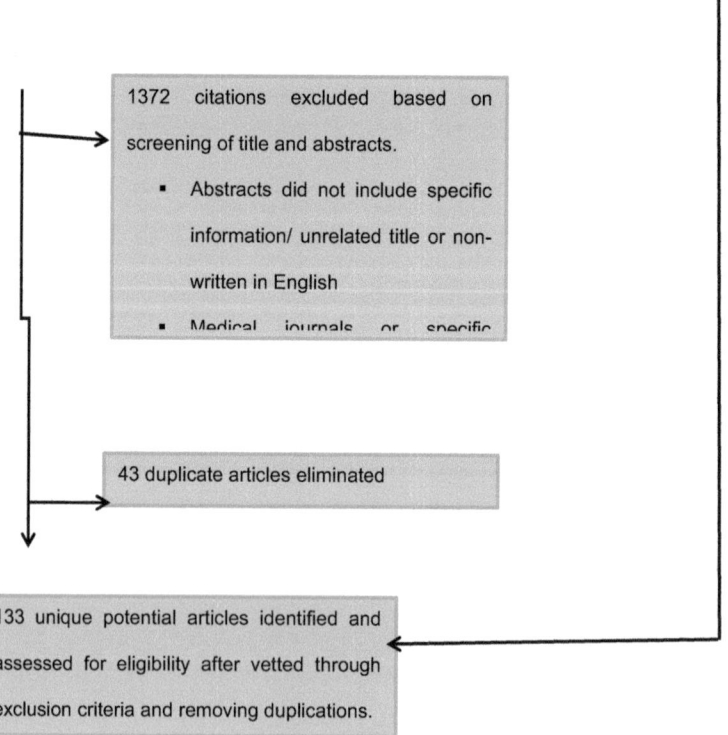

1385 articles identified from databases:

- o   64 in PubMed (Using Dementia" AND "Music Therapy" AND "Randomized Control trials"),)

- o   476 in CINAHL (Using Dementia" AND "Intervention" AND "Randomized Control

223 additional articles identified in reference lists using Google

1372 citations excluded based on screening of title and abstracts.
- Abstracts did not include specific information/ unrelated title or non-written in English
- Medical journals or specific

43 duplicate articles eliminated

133 unique potential articles identified and assessed for eligibility after vetted through exclusion criteria and removing duplications.

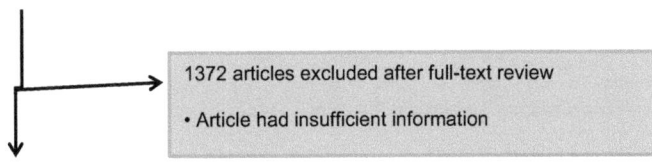

1372 articles excluded after full-text review

• Article had insufficient information

13 articles included in final review of RCTs

Table: Search Strategies:

Database Search	Search terms (Keywords)	Date assessed (2016-2017)	Number of studies identified with liberal screening of database	Excluded due to non-relevant data.	Studies for more detailed evaluation	Limit to the number of years, language and geographical area of study restrictions (6th Nov to 30th Dec, 2016)
CINAHL plus with full text	"Dementia" AND "Music Therapy" AND "Randomized Control trials"	6th Nov to 30th Dec	28	23	5	Limit to 10 years, English language only, place : UK
CINAHL plus with full text	"Dementia" AND "Intervention" AND "Randomized Control trials"	6th Nov to 30th Dec, 2016	447	439	8	Limit to 10 years, English language, only, place : UK

CINAHL plus with full text	"Dementia" AND "Cognitive therapy" AND "Randomized Control trials"	6th Nov to 30th Dec, 2016	01	0	01	Limit to 10 years, English language only, Place: UK
PubMed	"Dementia" AND "Music Therapy" AND "Randomized Control trials"	6th Nov to 30th Dec, 2016	67	63	4	Limit to 10 years, English language only, Place: UK
Cochrane Library	"Dementia" AND "Music Therapy" AND "Randomized Control trials"	6th Nov to 30th Dec, 2016	18	11	7	Limit to 10 years, English language only, Place: UK
ProQuest	"Dementia" AND "Music Therapy" AND	6th Nov to 30th Dec, 2016	23	18	5	Limit to 10 years, English language

	"Randomized Control trials"					only, Place: UK
VecNet	"Dementia" AND "Music Therapy" AND "Randomized Control trials"	6th Nov to 30th Dec, 2016	11	8	3	Limit to 10 years, English language only, Place: UK
Google scholar	"Dementia" AND "Music Therapy"	6th Nov to 30th Dec, 2016	223	216	7	Limit to 10 years, English language only, Place: UK
Database of Abstract of Reviews	"Dementia" AND "Cognitive therapy" AND "Randomized Control trials"	6th Nov to 30th Dec, 2016	567	480	87	Limit to 10 years, English language only, Place: UK
Total			1,385	1,258	127	
Relevant after reading the body of the		6th Nov, 2016 to	1,385	1,372	13	Limit to 10 years, English

article		15 Jan,				language
(Randomized		2017				only, Place:
Control trials)						UK

Ethical Approval Checklist:

University of Chester
Faculty of Health & Social Care
Research Ethics Sub-Committee

Please use when reviewing the application and complete ALL sections to ensure every aspect of the ethical review is considered. Please forward your review to hscethics@chester.ac.uk by the deadline.
Please note that this form will be sent out to the applicant. Please complete all sections.

Please indicate your opinion by placing a X or ✓ in the relevant box – You can cut and paste the symbols for ease:	Yes	No
Do you consider this to be for non-committee review?	✓	
Does this involve research abroad?		✓
Is this going to IRAS?		✓
Is this a clinical trial?		✓
Does this require subject specialist review?		✓

	General	Yes	No	N/A
1.1	Has the application form been received and completed appropriately and in full - written in English; all sections completed; date and version number included?	✓		
1.2	Has the applicant obtained all the necessary signatures?	✓		
1.3	Has a summary C.V. been provided for the Lead Researcher?			✓
1.4	Has a full list of references been provided?			✓
1.5	Has a participant information sheet been provided?			✓
1.6	Has a participant consent form been provided?			✓
1.7	Has a questionnaire (validated or non-validated) been provided?			✓
1.8	Have letters of invitation been provided?			✓
1.9	Have copies of recruitment advertisements been provided?			✓
1.10	Has written consent for use of facilities/commodities/other been provided?			✓

	Application Form	Yes	No	N/A
2.1	Do the titles suitably reflect the proposed research?	✓		
2.2	Does the applicant have suitable knowledge/experience to conduct the proposed research?	✓		
2.3	Is suitability of additional researchers/assistants acceptable?			✓
2.4	Is the suitability of the project supervisor acceptable?	✓		
2.5	Is there suitable justification for the relevance of the study, and has sufficient background information been provided?	✓		
2.6	Is the research design appropriate?	✓		
2.7	Is the sample size appropriate and, where applicable, justified by a statistical power calculation?			✓
2.8	Has the applicant sufficiently considered and addressed the potential benefits and risks of participation?			✓
2.9	Has the applicant clearly stated the method(s) proposed for identifying and recruiting potential participants?			✓
2.10	Has the applicant provided satisfactory justification for their inclusion and exclusion criteria?			✓
2.11	Has the applicant sufficiently considered and addressed the potential ethical issues related to participation in the study?			✓
2.12	Has the applicant explained clearly how consent will be obtained?			✓
2.13	Has the applicant sufficiently addressed issues regarding confidentiality: participant integrity; privacy and protection of data?			✓
2.14	Has the applicant provided details of measures to be taken to ensure participants are free to withdraw from the study without adverse effects?			✓
2.15	Has the applicant sufficiently indicated any special measures to be taken to safeguard the interests of any identified vulnerable groups?			✓
2.16	Has the applicant provided sufficient details of the methodology for data collection?	✓		
2.17	Has the applicant provided sufficient details of the methodology for data analysis?	✓		

	Participant Information Sheet (where applicable)	Yes	No	N/A
3.1	Has the applicant clearly identified protocols and timescales to participants?			✓
3.2	Has the applicant addressed all issues relating to confidentiality?			✓
3.3	Has the applicant included details of a relevant contact in the event of something going wrong during the study?			✓
3.4	Has the applicant provided University contact details for themselves, as opposed to personal details?			✓
3.5	Is the documentation free from grammatical or typographical errors?			✓

Consent Form (where applicable)	Yes	No	N/A
4.1	Have all the relevant consents been requested, such as consent to be tape recorded; consent to be contacted for a follow-up interview etc.?			✓
4.2	Is the documentation free from grammatical or typographical errors?			✓

Do you have any further comments you wish to make?

Yes ☑   No ☐

Please expand on the points above to which you have responded 'No', and make any additional comments in the space below, particularly in relation to additional documentation not specified above.

Please write your comments directly to the applicant.

Leader Reviewer
This is a systematic literature review and as a desktop exercise, apart from the usual need for rigour, does not present any other ethical issues

Second Reviewer
I agree with the comments of the lead reviewer and it is clear that this is a systematic review of the literature.

Which category applies here? Please indicate your decision by inserting a X or ✓ - cut and paste the symbol for ease.					
Ethical Approval Granted	✓	Points to address		Full Resubmission Needed	

Appendix 14: Deaths due to Dementia in 2012:

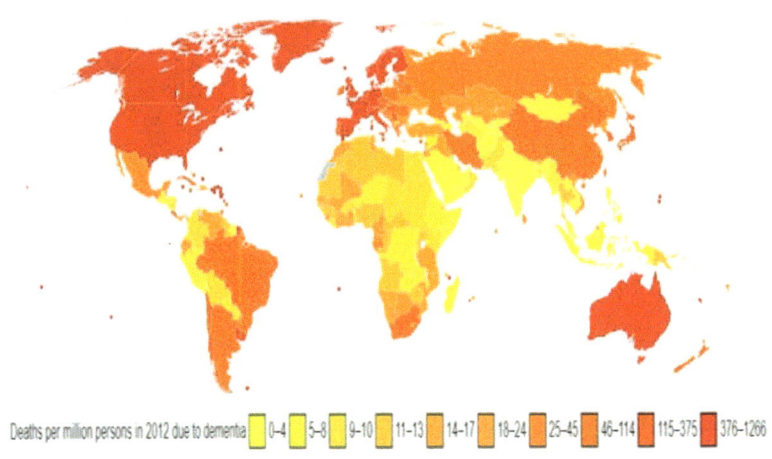

Deaths per million persons in 2012 due to dementia ▮0–4 ▮5–8 ▮9–10 ▮11–13 ▮14–17 ▮18–24 ▮25–45 ▮46–114 ▮115–375 ▮376–1266

Literature Review: Example:

Database (searched 11.2.14)	Initial number of hits	After review of titles	Combined hits after duplicates removed	Combined hits after review of abstracts and content	Total hits retained	After exclusion of literature reviews and "concept papers"
JSTOR	6	6	57	28	46	8 Anecdotal/case studies
Proquest	149	35				5 Autobiographical
Psycinfo	268	33		Citation/ reference search additional		13 Interview
ScienceDirect	40	6		18		5 Proxy

Figure 11: Buggey, T. (2007, Summer).. Diagram. Journal of Positive Behavior Interventions, 9(3), 151. Retrieved December 14, 2007, from Academic Search Premier database.

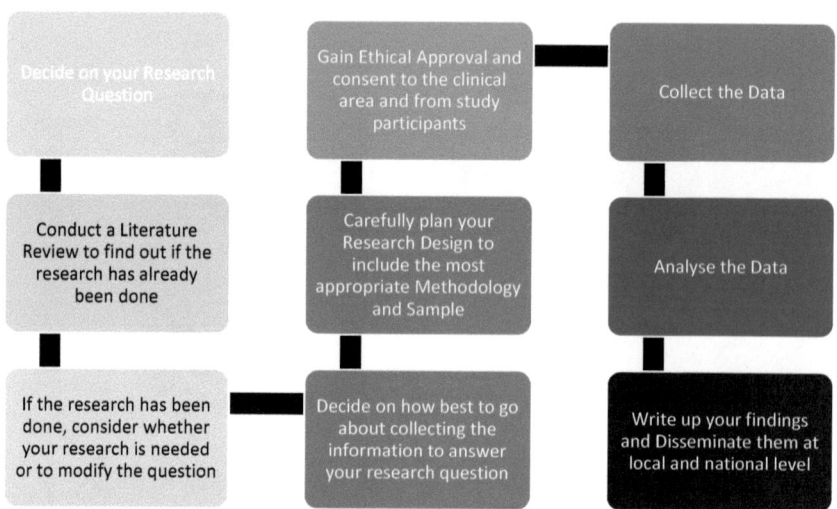

Figure 12: Research Process (Watson R & Keady (2008)

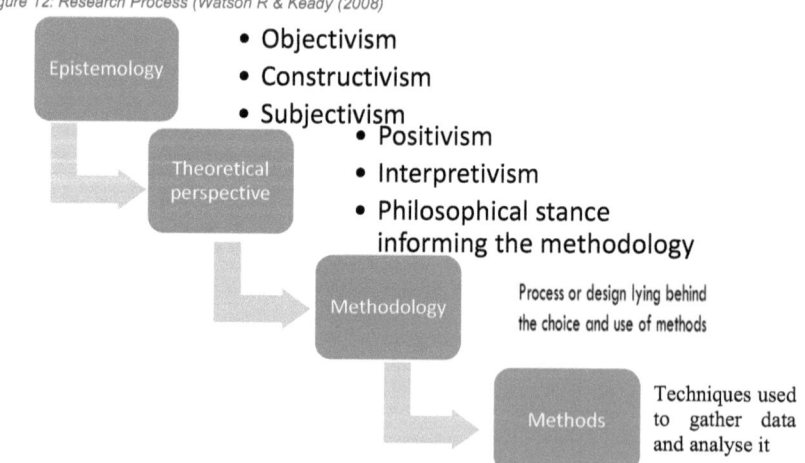

- Objectivism
- Constructivism
- Subjectivism
  - Positivism
  - Interpretivism
  - Philosophical stance informing the methodology

Process or design lying behind the choice and use of methods

Techniques used to gather data and analyse it

Figure 13 RESEARCH STAGES (Watson R & Keady (2008)

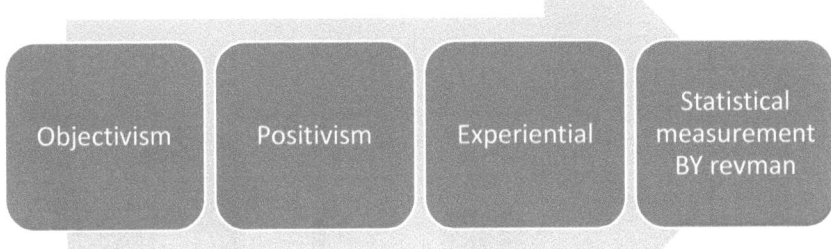

Figure 14: Research Steps (Followed) (Watson R & Keady (2008)

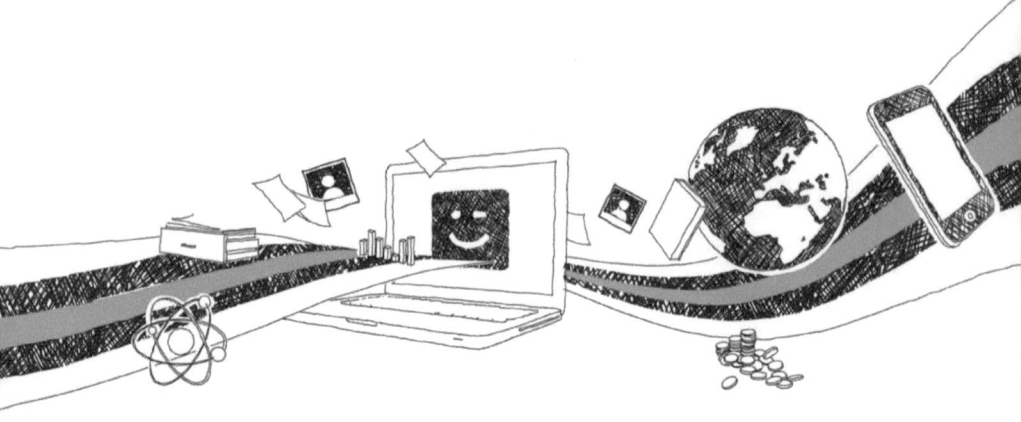
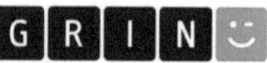